CURING
INFERTILITY

WITH ANCIENT CHINESE MEDICINE

CURING INFERTILITY

WITH ANCIENT CHINESE MEDICINE

HOW TO BECOME PREGNANT AND HEALTHY WITH THE HUNYUAN METHOD

YARON SEIDMAN, DAOM
FOREWORD BY KAROL J. CHACHO, MD

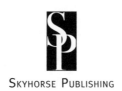

Skyhorse Publishing

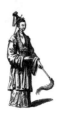

Skyhorse Publishing books may be purchased in bulk at special discounts for sales promotion, corporate gifts, fund-raising, or educational purposes. Special editions can also be created to specifications. For details, contact the Special Sales Department, Skyhorse Publishing, 307 West 36th Street, 11th Floor, New York, NY 10018 or info@skyhorsepublishing.com.

Skyhorse® and Skyhorse Publishing® are registered trademarks of Skyhorse Publishing, Inc.®, a Delaware corporation.

Visit our website at www.skyhorsepublishing.com.

10 9 8 7 6 5 4 3 2 1

Library of Congress Cataloging-in-Publication Data is available on file.

ISBN: 978-1-62087-585-8

Printed in the United States of America

For my mother and father, who by making the correct choices in life, taught me the traditional values necessary to lead my children down a path toward health, well-being, and fulfillment.

CONTENTS

• • • • • • • •

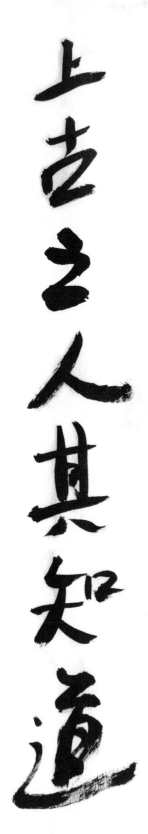

上吉之人其知道

FOREWORD

• • • • • • • •

Like most aspects of modern medicine, the treatment of infertility has become a "high-tech" process. Acronyms such as IVF (in-vitro fertilization), ICSI (intracytoplasmic sperm injection) and PGD (pre-implantation genetic diagnosis) have become all too familiar to couples considering or undergoing infertility treatment. In most areas of medicine, high-tech advances constitute major strides in the conquest of disease. With infertility, these advances have also made treatment a cold, clinical process rather than the natural process that most couples anticipate.

The first IVF baby was born in 1978 and the process became clinically available in the mid-1980s. Prior to that, reproductive endocrinologists using proven tecŸiques helped many infertile couples achieve pregnancy. Although some of those tecŸiques, such as surgery to correct pelvic problems, were certainly clinical, many were more natural, involving hormone treatments, tracking of the menstrual cycle and properly timed intercourse. Most of these tecŸiques are still available today but have fallen by the wayside thanks to the contemporary approach of high-tech infertility treatments.

This clinicalization of infertility treatment has also extended into the realm of traditional Chinese medicine, a discipline where the personal touch has always been held sacred. Because of peer-reviewed research, certain ancient Chinese tecŸiques have gradually been accepted by Western infertility medicine. Most notably, IVF pregnancy rates have been shown to improve with acupuncture. Consequently, many current practitioners of traditional Chinese medicine have geared their practices toward these findings and learn only those aspects of eastern tecŸiques that relate directly to IVF or other Western treatments. They do not study many of the ancient Chinese remedies and treatments that for thousands of years have helped couples conceive.

In this book, Yaron Seidman explores in depth this loss of traditional tecŸiques of infertility treatment and discusses alternatives to the contemporary approach.

He proposes the adoption of an innovative combination of the best of noninvasive Western reproductive medicine and the best of traditional Chinese medicine backed up, if necessary, by modern high-tech treatments. The majority of infertile couples would undoubtedly prefer this combination of natural tecŸiques versus going directly to drugs, injections, and plastic cups.

Karol Chacho, M.D.,
*Board Certified Infertility Specialist
and Reproductive Endocrinologist*

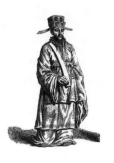

PREFACE

• • • • • • •

Chinese medicine, known as the "science of time," preceded modern science by at least 3,000 years. In *Curing Infertility with Ancient Chinese Medicine* we will travel the path of this ancient discipline step by step to discover its genius. Though primarily intended for infertility patients, the book is also aimed at Modern Chinese medical practitioners, most of whom lack any training in the classical ways.

To truly grasp the essence of Ancient Chinese medicine, we must leave modern thinking patterns behind. If viewed from the perspective of Western medicine, the discipline's meaning and enormous value will be missed entirely. If approached with an open mind, an amazing world will open.

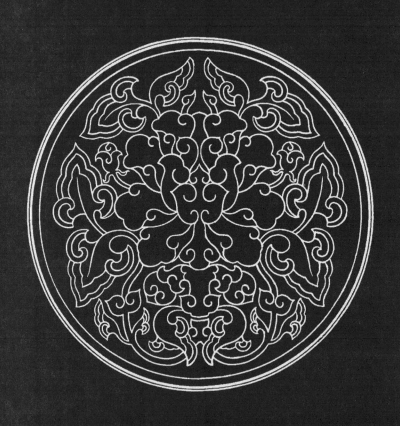

AUTHOR'S FOREWORD

· · · · · · · · · · · · · ·

I took fertility drugs at the beginning of this IVF cycle, as instructed by my reproductive endocrinologist. The doctor harvested fourteen perfectly healthy eggs, out of which twelve fertilized. We did genetic testing to determine which embryos were the best quality. The doctor transferred three of these best quality embryos ... and then we waited anxiously until the scheduled blood test just to find out that the pregnancy didn't take.

This story and others are commonplace at my Hunyuan Centers in Connecticut. We see women who repeatedly try In Vitro Fertilization and fail to conceive. In most cases, the doctor cannot explain what went wrong. Everything was "going according to plan" and yet in the end, nothing happened.

As the founder of the Hunyuan Method, my main concern is with the patient's health. I know from experience that when a woman is truly healthy, she can conceive and maintain a pregnancy naturally without artificial help.

As of yet, general knowledge of healthy natural conception is at best unsatisfactory. The average fertility patient is told to try "naturally" for six to twelve months, and if unsuccessful, to immediately proceed to drugs, invasive tests, and/or surgical procedures. Sometimes treatment is recommended after just one month of trying naturally. Yet, the side effects of these treatments are many and the success rate is low.

Becoming truly healthy before attempting to conceive naturally optimizes a woman's chances for conception and will often prevent endless expensive fertility treatments. We have all experienced illness and disease when our bodies simply did not work well. Optimum health is not only important for the mother's reproductive capacity and safety, it is also significant when it comes to the baby's development.

In the world of modern fertility treatments, health is often ignored. Stimulating the ovaries with drugs, or removing fibroids and fallopian tubes, does not make a woman healthy. Removal of eggs for fertilization, followed by replacement in the uterus, does not make a woman healthy. In fact, side effects I have seen in my patients taking fertility medications include hot flashes, abdominal distension, cysts, menstrual irregularities, elevated FSH levels, emotional breakdowns, back pain, heart palpitations, and insomnia.

If you are at all familiar with Chinese medicine, the method to attain fertility presented here will no doubt seem very foreign. It is different from what most Chinese medicine doctors practice today. It explains "Health" from a "Hunyuan Method" perspective. "Hunyuan" is my term for Classical Chinese medicine, developed by the ancients, which is now practiced by very few. In this discipline, the doctor's first calling is to educate and inform his patients on how to stay healthy. It is different from, and often completely contradictory to, "Modern Chinese medicine," which, like Western medicine, is more concerned with treating symptoms.

Although I do not believe in taking most pharmaceutical drugs, I have a great admiration for Western medicine. Primarily occupied with symptoms and their instant elimination, Western medicine does so with great conviction and success. When a drug is intended to stimulate the ovaries, for example, it does so without hesitation.

On the other hand, my admiration for Classical Chinese medicine rises out of its swiftness in eliminating the *root* cause of an illness. I can think of endless examples to support this notion, but one that I will share involves a forty-two-year-old patient with a sinus infection that lasted for three months. She took three rounds of strong antibiotics, and although her symptoms lessened after each round, the symptoms continued to return within one to two days. When she came to see me, she complained of exhaustion, relentless headaches, and constant coughing-up of green phlegm. I composed a Classical Chinese medicine formula made out of three herbs. When she returned the following week, she reported that after drinking the first cup of herbal tea, her head cleared within two hours, and by the next morning, her symptoms were gone. Two months later, the patient conceived naturally and at the time of this writing is eight months pregnant with no complications.

Modern Chinese medicine does not favor herbal formulas— instead, the use of acupuncture is more common for treating infertility cases. Although modern studies suggest that placing acupuncture needles in a few predetermined points can improve IVF (In Vitro Fetilization) success rates, these treatments are not nearly as effective as the Classical Chinese herbal formulas.

"Health" is a relative concept. Although we may not be in optimum health, we feel healthy because we tend to compare ourselves to others who are less healthy. I will explain in this book what "health" should and shouldn't look like, and how to improve, remedy, and preserve it. Most importantly, I will show how improving your health can help you become pregnant.

Statistics show that 14 percent of all couples in the United States suffer from infertility. This translates to millions and millions of people, and hundreds of millions of dollars spent on infertility treatments. It is my hope that this book will allow the reader to make a better, or at least a more informed, choice as to what course of action to take with fertility treatments. Hopefully, the reader will realize that sometimes the fastest way is not necessarily the easiest way, or the right way.

The one comment I hear most often from my patients is "I wish I had known about you earlier." What would happen if women with infertility issues turned to the Hunyuan method before turning to Western medicine? Although there's no definitive answer to this question, I am certain that thousands of childless couples would have known the joy of parenting.

Yaron Seidman, L.Ac., DAOM
Greenwich, Connecticut

術起食飲有節

居有常不妄作勞

故能形與神俱而

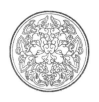

···· 1 ····

GIVE THE ANCIENTS A CHANCE

"Salad causes cancer," was something I was surprised to hear during a lecture by a well-known nutritionist. Of course, she wasn't referring to the vegetables in the salad, but to the chemical-laden dressings most Americans pour on top of them. The lesson was that lack of knowledge about ingredients could lead to disease. The same is true with infertility. With the right knowledge, infertility can often be avoided. Without the right knowledge, infertility will prevail.

"The sages knew how to live in harmony with nature. They lived to be one hundred years old but their bodies never declined and they looked as if they were only fifty years old," opens *The Yellow Emperor Inner Classics*, a 2,500-year-old treatise that forms the essence of Chinese medicine.

The methods of these sages, transmitted over generations, provide a stark contrast to today's prevailing notion that new is better than old when it comes to the practice of medicine. We cling to the false beliefs that our methods are increasingly efficient and that previous generations knew less than we do.

I am convinced that this idealization of what is new and "advanced" contributes to many of the diseases from which we suffer today. It is certainly a major cause of infertility, a condition that was far less common when medical procedures were less complicated. Modern science gives us a new set of options that can actually cause more illness and leaves many more people living on drugs. Many pharmaceuticals are known to produce debilitating side effects and long-term deterioration. I often hear claims such as "This drug will cure your high cholesterol, but it might lead to liver problems in the future." And fertility drug treatments are no exception; there is a marked deterioration in the health of a woman taking fertility drugs as an increased number of women suffer from infertility, miscarriages, and/or pregnancy complications.

Originally, I accepted the theory that the present infertility boom was caused by the trend of women focusing on their careers before having a family. However, after treating many hundreds of "infertility patients," I am certain that choosing to have a child later in life is not the only cause and perhaps not even the most important. In fact, many of my patients are in their twenties, and statistics show that women are now experiencing infertility at a younger age than previously.

GIVING UP MODERN PREJUDICES

To understand classical Chinese medicine, the reader must attempt to remain nonjudgmental until completing this book in order to avoid distraction by modern prejudice. You must be able to think beyond both Western medical science and modern Chinese medical science in order to see the flaws in those systems and to see how these two disciplines have robbed Chinese medicine of its essence.

THE HIGH AND THE LOW

In ancient China, an individual's health was thought to be more precious than a thousand gold bars. The ancient Chinese thought that human life was created out of the interaction between heaven and earth. Furthermore, the harmonization of heaven and earth was thought to equal the prolonging of one's health. They felt that with healthy people living long lives, the natural cycle of birth and rebirth would go on forever, exactly like heaven and earth go on forever, birthing and rebirthing day after day and year after year.

The Chinese culture has spawned many brilliant physicians over its thousands of years of history. One such physician was Zhang Ji who lived during the second century AD. In the early years of his practice, he warned a duke that if he neglected to take a particular herbal formula, he would lose his eyebrows in twenty years and subsequently die a terrible death. The duke, a doctor himself, laughed it off, unable to believe in a diagnosis twenty years in advance. Nevertheless, twenty years later, the Duke's eyebrows fell off, and within three months he fell ill and died in great pain.

Zhang Ji's reputation grew until he was famous far and wide. Adopting the pen name Zhang Zhongjing, he wrote a book that is considered one of the four classics of Chinese medicine for the past 2,000 years and provides a foundation for the discipline.

Zhang Zhongjing and other physicians like him were centuries ahead of their time. They can be likened to Albert Einstein, whose theories about space and black holes in the universe still evade comprehension by many scientists today. Zhang and other ancient geniuses established the rules for harmonizing the body with nature, paving the way for long life and health. As healers, they were dedicated to the long-term benefit of the patient, and when they prescribed herbs, it was to heal for a lifetime, hence Zhang's ability to see his patient's condition twenty years ahead. Because of this long-term view, Zhang is referred to in Chinese medicine as a "high practitioner."

Unfortunately, this principle can be difficult to follow. Understanding the impact of one's actions for many years to come is not an easy feat. This gave birth to the "low-level practitioner," who was occupied with short-term success in alleviating symptoms. According to *The Yellow Emperor* in his first volume, *Plain Questions*, a low-level practitioner treats disease with a standard formula, while high-level practitioners treat disease by analyzing the situation and then coming up with an appropriate solution.

BRINGING BACK THE TRUE CHINESE MEDICINE

The popularity of acupuncture has long been increasing in the Western world, largely because practitioners and acupuncture schools have made an effort to integrate into mainstream Western medicine. While this is very encouraging on some levels, it also pushes the practice of acupuncture toward the Western medicine model of treating symptoms, and away from the Chinese medicine concern with long-lasting health benefits.

This is particularly true when it comes to treatments for infertility. Most acupuncture practitioners who embrace Western medicine's endocrinology-related issues give up traditional Chinese principles to follow the mainstream model of health. Unfortunately, this means that traditional Chinese medicine is all but extinct.

Ironically, in Zhang Zhongjing's time, a similar situation had developed. In the introduction to *Shang Hanlun*, Zhang writes:

"I always admired the diagnosis and skills of the talented doctors of the past. It is strange that the doctors today are not cautious with medicine and herbs and their research of the herbal prescriptions is not thorough. They pursue on their tiptoes glory and power, their service is for fame and profit alone. They worship the tail end of the discipline and they forget about its essence. They magnify the outer shell and forget about the inner core. If the skin is not there, how can the body hair be at peace?

"Doctors everywhere are losing their heads and can't reach enlightenment. They do not cherish 'life' as if it were a benign affair, so how can they talk about fame and power? Their diagnosis can only be partial and they can't see the entire picture. This is called viewing the patient through a peephole."

Zhang believed that to be truly effective, practitioners had to be immersed in the classics until it was part of their being. He also explained that to love the body and to honestly help patients, the practitioner must first learn about himself.

BELIEVING IN THE PATIENT AND HER BODY

Western doctors whose IVF treatments fail are prone to blame the patient, generally because she is "too old," whether that means she's thirty or forty-six. When my patients fail to become pregnant with the Hunyuan Method, I view it as my failure.

It is of utmost importance to have total faith in the patient and her body. Western medicine believes that an organ or body function that fails cannot recover by itself and needs intervention, such as with IVF. Chinese medicine always believes that the patient's body can recover its functions on its own.

This difference in perspective lies in our different approach to thinking about the future. In Western thought, when the future is uncertain, most people believe that the outcome will be negative. This engenders a sense of safety in that Westerners already know something bad is going to happen, and thus cannot be surprised by it. In Asia, and especially in China, the approach has been quite different. The Chinese feel content over whatever the future brings, that nature is on their side, and that if they follow nature, the future will always be bright.

In Western medicine, if there is any question about a patient's condition and the doctor has to decide if the patient is ill or healthy, the tendency is to opt for illness. If the choice is to medicate or not, the decision will usually be to medicate. This is because it is "better" to pronounce someone ill and be wrong than to pronounce someone "well" and be wrong. It is believed that prescribing medication that is not necessary will simply be wasteful, but not harmful.

Extended to the world of infertility treatments, Western doctors start with the assumption that the woman has little chance of becoming pregnant. Expectations are lowered so if the patient does become pregnant, the doctor becomes a hero. In Chinese medicine, it is believed that only nature can decide who is fertile and who is not, and if the patient is healthy and in tune with nature, there's a good chance pregnancy will occur. Doctors cannot make it happen.

My experience shows that believing in nature always leads to a brighter future. Many patients in my practice have experienced it firsthand. They believed in their own fertility and they became pregnant naturally.

When a patient comes to see me, it isn't necessary for me to shatter her dreams and cause her to sink into despair, fearing the future. I encourage her and boost her confidence because it feels good to be treated with Chinese medicine. After every acupuncture session the patient feels invigorated. After every week of herbs, the patient feels more vital. If nothing else, excellent health is always achieved.

Infertility patients seeking help from Chinese medicine should seek out a practitioner specializing in Classical Chinese medicine. Patients seeking help via Western medicine should visit a reproductive endocrinologist (RE). Combining Western medicine with acupuncture by a Modern Chinese medicine practitioner, or doing IVF with a Western doctor specializing in acupuncture, should be avoided. The disciplines simply do not mix. Western medicine can help if you use the right specialist RE, and Chinese medicine can help if you use a classically trained practitioner specializing in infertility.

Many women have become pregnant with the Hunyuan Method despite the fact that their Western doctor has assured them there was no possible way to become pregnant naturally because of their age. As *The Yellow Emperor* says, "The ones who live by nature, their body will be as if they are half their age and for those who live in contradiction to nature their body will be as if they are twice their age."

Certainly age counts, but so does health, including what you eat, how you sleep, how much stress you endure, and what chemicals and drugs you are consuming.

It is time for each patient to become individually enlightened. I believe that many "infertile" couples will succeed naturally if only they will give themselves the chance. Patients must not let themselves be discouraged into IVF.

WESTERN MEDICINE – THE GOOD AND THE UGLY

In the past one hundred years, Western medicine has made enormous progress. Today's tecŸology and equipment for advanced diagnosis and surgery is indeed remarkable. However, along with success and advance there are some pitfalls as well. Sometimes power and conviction lead to a "my-way-or-the-highway" attitude.

Jerome Groopman, a cancer specialist, delivers a sharp and coherent critique of medicine's mistaken direction. In his book, *How Doctors Think*, he writes that approximately 15 percent of diagnoses are inaccurate, and that in medical schools, students are rarely taught to ask how an error could have taken place, let alone how it might be avoided in the future.

Most Western doctors are unaware of their mistakes. Even if patients remain unwell, no systematic effort is made to find out where doctors may have gone wrong. This is partly because most doctors believe there is no alternative to the treatment they have prescribed.

DRUGS AND POLITICS

In a survey of over 1,600 American physicians, nine out of ten reported a relationship with a pharmaceutical company. The benefits they received ranged from drug samples to tickets for sporting events, speaking honorariums, and payments in exchange for persuading patients to join clinical trials. The pressure of increasingly aggressive marketing tactics by the pharmaceutical companies only adds to a climate of endless misunderstanding. Most doctors receive information about new drugs directly from pharmaceutical representatives. Rarely do they personally investigate what is known about a drug. This dependency on biased information leaves doctors improperly equipped to make balanced judgments about which drugs to prescribe and when they should prescribe them.

We have all witnessed the great number of medications recalled by the Food and Drug Administration over the years, and even more where warnings have been issued. When it comes to fertility drugs, some medications prescribed by Western doctors are not approved by the FDA for fertility treatment. It is therefore imperative that infertility patients about to begin drug therapy research the short- and long-term safety of the medication they will be taking. In my opinion, if no studies can be found that guarantee the safety of a particular medication, then it must be considered unsafe.

MODERN CHINESE MEDICINE: TOO WESTERN FOR ITS OWN GOOD

Several years ago I was introduced to another acupuncturist who specializes in administering acupuncture in conjunction with IVF treatments. Although she would prefer to prescribe herbs as well, Western medical doctors did not allow for that. She concluded that the acupuncture treatment was effective on its own. "Does it matter what way the patient gets pregnant?" she asked me. "We only want to get them pregnant."

I believe that it does matter. Achieving good health, becoming pregnant, and giving birth to a healthy baby is preferable to simply becoming pregnant. Unfortunately, many practitioners don't understand the difference, and many actually believe that it is impossible for an infertility patient to become pregnant using Chinese medicine without IVF. I believe this is largely a result of ignorance of Chinese medicine classics by many practitioners. According to *The Yellow Emperor*, women can get pregnant until the age of forty-nine, and if they are following the Dao Eastern philosophical nature of the universe, even older.

I believe that Chinese medicine practitioners should practice true Chinese medicine. Working in conjunction with each other, we can move closer to Western medicine.

THE WISDOM OF THE ANCIENTS

For generations, the human species created dietary habits to fit into their environment and resources. Certain foods lead to survival while others did not. Each culture developed a some-what different diet according to climate, traditions, resources and needs. For example, dairy products were widely used in European cultures but hardly used in eastern Asian cultures with resulting biological consequences. To truly know the correct foods we should be consuming, we must take into consideration the season, our location on the planet, as well as our ancestry.

Unfortunately, modern society has moved away from this wisdom. Although we believe we live healthier lives than previous generations, we find ourselves debilitated by more illness. The public is under constant bombardment by an overwhelming degree of misinformation about what is healthy and what is not, leading to tremendous confusion.

When patients first come to me, I often hear such statements as"my grandmother used to cook with lard (fat), ate a lot of butter, and lived to be ninety-five. She was never sick and she had five kids. I am eating 'healthy'—a lot of salad and fat-free dairy—and I can't get pregnant."

From a fertility standpoint, the grandmother's diet is in many ways better than her granddaughter's. Most patients I treat come to me absolutely convinced that they are eating very healthily, when in fact their diets are very poor, at least for achieving pregnancy.

SHELF LIFE – MORE IMPORTANT THAN HUMAN LIFE

Enemy number one, of course, is the processed food manufactured by huge corporations looking at their own bottom line rather than the public's best interest. Shelf life becomes more important than human life, and lowering the cost of production is more important than keeping the ingredients healthy. Chemicals are added to preserve fresŸess and the public doesn't seem to care about what that means when it comes to their bodies.

The centralized production of food is also anathema to good health. In order to move from production to distribution center, which can be 2,000 miles away, food must be processed to last as long as possible. Glitches and accidents in manufacturing can impact an entire nation, as evidenced by the e-coli outbreak resulting from centralized spinach distribution. Even the word "organic" no longer has the same meaning. More health conscious individuals are purchasing food grown locally in their area.

(NOT SO) NATURAL SUPPLEMENTS

Millions of Americans spend billions of dollars per year on dietary supplements, believing that they cannot get all the vitamins they need from the food they purchase. Although it is true that many of today's supermarkets offer only processed, modified, centralized, and depleted food, it is incorrect to assume that supplements will be a substitute for healthy food. They will never replace milk, meat, fresh fruits and vegetables, or clean air and water. Supplements are not natural. They were not made by nature. One will not find a multivitamin pill growing on a tree.

Despite the excessive use of supplements the American public has purchased over the past several decades, we are burdened with an increase in debilitating diseases such as cancer, heart disease, diabetes, asthma, allergies and infertility. Is this progress? I believe we need to get our vitamins from the proper food—the food our forefathers ate—that is not found on a supermarket shelf.

I rely on the ancient wisdom for my health. My mother didn't take pills, nor did my grandmother or my great-grandmother, and it goes back like this for endless generations. Why should I break this tradition by taking supplements?

Once a month I drive out to a farm in rural Connecticut to purchase a monthly supply of chickens for my family. The product is not certified organic, but in the farmer's words is simply "raised the way the Lord intended." When I visit local farms to purchase chicken, milk, meat, and produce, I feel reassured that I am taking proper care of my family by providing them with excellent food, while also supporting the farmers who make that possible.

Flowing with nature is far preferable to conquering it. Genuinely healthy food heals people and makes them fertile. Depleted food and supplements do not.

LIFESTYLE – A CRUCIAL COMPONENT IN FERTILITY

The Chinese medicine classics emphasize the need to understand Yin and Yang to stay in balance by not doing too much or too little, as well as to follow the Dao (often spelled "Tao"), which means the harmony of nature. The three primary areas where modern society does not follow either principle are work, sleep, and stimulation.

The most acute problem of our modern lifestyle is our excessive work schedule. According to Chinese medicine guidelines, one should wake up at sunrise, plow his field through the early morning hours, and then sit under the tree and rest for the remainder of the day.

Today's work habits are considerably different. Our bodies are exhausted day in and day out. *The Yellow Emperor's Plain Questions* says that to bear children, the kidneys must be full of energy, but when we work too hard or too long, our kidneys are depleted of that energy. Patients often tell me that they start the day at 7 A.M. and finish work at 9 or 10 P.M. True, we sometimes feel energized when we are wrapped up in our work. We must understand, however, that the hard work is not what is creating the energy. Our bodies are extracting the extra energy from our kidneys.

Modern fertility drugs exhaust the body further. Working hard and using fertility drugs simultaneously is tantamount to the body pulling in two different directions. Sometimes the situation is even more difficult because the cost of the fertility drugs requires us to work even harder. Under such circumstances, the kidney's Yang energy is drained.

If you hope to become pregnant, the first step is to work less and spend more relaxing time in nature. This is following the Dao of nature.

With the invention of electricity and light, our sleeping habits have gradually changed. *The Yellow Emperor* classic describes in detail how to harmonize with nature by following the patterns of the sun, hence sleeping more in winter and less in summer. When the body follows the harmony of nature, infertility will not set in before the age of forty-nine. But if one works constantly and routinely stays up until 2 A.M., the body will not have the chance it needs to do its job.

Jessica had tried everything: IUIs, IVFs, and even Chinese medicine but nothing worked. Yaron Seidman says that after Jessica's friend became pregnant with the help of the Hunyuan Method, she grew curious. Yaron says that at first she was skeptical, but after learning the difference between ancient and modern Chinese medicine, she decided to give ancient Chinese medicine a try. She conceived within three months. Jessica says that when she took the herbal formulas of the ancient method, it felt so different than the other modern formulas had before. She says that she felt so energetic and alive almost immediately, not to mention that it helped her conceive too.

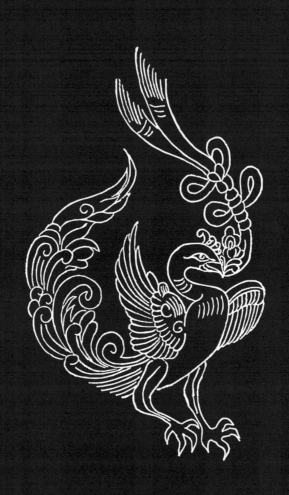

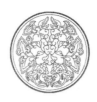

2

UNDERSTANDING CHINESE MEDICINE

For centuries Chinese physicians explored energy relationships between humans and the universe. In the first 1,500 years of Chinese medicine's development, this metascience was dominant. Significant concepts such as Yin and Yang and the five elements took shape and solidified. However, in the following dynasties, this trend changed and new theories came into place as physicians began explaining phenomena from a scientific standpoint.

It is important to return to a metascience understanding of Chinese medicine, because it is impossible to create effective herbal formulas and acupuncture protocols without this perspective. Although modern Chinese medicine, like Western medicine, can often relieve symptoms, it works contrary to the Chinese rule of curing the root of the illness.

It is important to understand there is a connection between all aspects of our energy, and that any action we take has an impact on our health and fertility. It is not only the ovaries or uterus lining problems that are related to fertility. What we eat, how we sleep, and how we medicate all impact different aspects of our energy.

This approach can best be understood in terms of the concept of Yin and Yang, which demonstrates how seemingly opposite or contrary forces are interconnected and interdependent in the natural world.

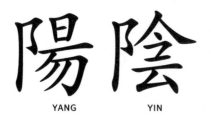

YANG   YIN

The right section of the Yang character has three parts. The upper part is a sun in the sky. The middle part is the line under the sun, which represents the earth. The third part is the lines under the earth, representing the sun's rays of light and warmth. In its entirety, this side of the character stands for energy, or the outdoors.

The same can be said for the right character which is the Yin character. The upper part is the roof of a house. The middle part is a person sitting in the house. The bottom is the steam coming out of cooked rice or cooked food. It represents the Yin energy, which is indoors, and has to do with our physical body or with physical matter. The bottom represents the presence of energy which is hot in nature but is not coming directly from the sun. Instead it comes from elements that were derived from the earth with the sun's help like rice, water, and firewood.

When we compare both characters, we see that we are dealing with two different states of energy. In the Yang character, the sun's rays go downwards, while in the Yin character the steam is going upwards. Yang has less matter and more energy, and gives us the force for life. Yin is the opposite. It has more matter and less energy, giving us the energy associated with matter, needed for life. In Chinese medicine, living physical matter, such as body tissues, bones, and muscles, is in a state of condensed energy. The Yang energy, however, is energy we cannot see. It is physical matter but it contains energy within.

Both Yin and Yang characters have a section on the left side representing a hill or a mound. The hill is where the earth is swollen like a pregnant woman, and is the place where the earth is growing closer to the heavens. It is a symbol of heaven and earth exchanging energies, and of life and future generations.

24

The hill to the left summarizes the characters of Yin and Yang. Whether it is physical living matter or invisible life's energy, both represent the exchange of heaven and earth. Both are living and needed for life. The life force, whether outside or inside the body, is warm. Therefore, the Yang energy and the Yin matter must all contain this warmth, which is the root of life.

MEDICINE OF "TIME"

Chinese medicine at its core explores only one concept: time. This is very different than modern Chinese medicine and Western medicine, which explore space.

The sages realized the unity of things. Everything in our world can be pulled back into unison under one concept. *The Yellow Emperor* explains, "As to exploring Yin and Yang, you can take ten and make it a hundred, you can take a thousand and make it ten thousand, and you can separate it in that manner endlessly. However, in pulling it back together, it is only one Yin and Yang."

"Time" is what allows us to understand this unity. In Chinese medicine, the concept of "time" goes far beyond how we conceive it today. To grasp time, we must gradually recalibrate our thinking process to match that of the sages.

The Yellow Emperor explains, "The ancient sages knew the Dao, they followed Yin and Yang, they harmonized with the ancient arts and numbers, their diet had rules, their sleeping and living habits were regulated, and they didn't labor for nothing. Their bodies united with their spirit, they fulfilled their heavenly years, lived to be a hundred and then they departed."

The progression from conception to birth, childhood, adulthood and into decline and death represents a single line of time. *The Yellow Emperor* calls it the "heavenly years." The genius of the ancient sages is their understanding of the meaning of this "stretch of time," the true meaning of life.

The sages believed that life, like time, is intangible. You can't grasp it, box it, shape it, or calculate it. However, you can know its Dao, or the laws and rules that compose it. *The Yellow Emperor* explains that the rules of life or the rules of "time" follow Yin and Yang.

When one understands the rules of Yin and Yang, lifestyle, diet, sleeping, and work all change accordingly. When we understand the stretch of time we call life, or the stretch of life we call time, there is no other truth. The material world becomes invisible, a new realm of time opens up before us. Time, or the "heavenly years," is the only thing that matters.

Entering this Chinese medicine world, we find nothing more precious than time and nothing more precious than life. We do not own our lives nor do we own the stretch of time we are allocated by heaven. However, it is our responsibility as humans to live our heavenly years to their fullest extent. Thus it is our responsibility to understand life and how to keep it going all the way to the end. We have to know the Dao. We have to understand Yin and Yang.

In reality, "time" goes far beyond our lifetime. It extends to the heavenly years of our children, grandchildren, and endless generations thereafter. That the sages knew the Dao of heavenly years explains that they understood the significance of not only their own lives, but rather the heavenly years for billions of people over many thousands of years to come.

Although we have made great progress in science and technology, this signifies an advance solely in "space," and has concurrently brought about a retreat in our understanding of "time."

When modern science uses "time," the world of energy opens up. This is why there is a renaissance in China and around the world of classical Chinese medicine and research into "time" and "life." Doctors, mathematicians, and scientists are all beginning to ponder these questions of life once more. People are starting to ask questions such as "Is this drug really good for me? Is food sprayed with pesticides safe? Should I move to a place where there is cleaner air?"

INTRODUCING YIN AND YANG

The concept of time, as put forth by the sages, has different patterns representing different aspects of Yin and Yang. When a patient is sick or infertile, the practitioner's job is to identify which pattern of Yin and Yang is not working properly. This is called differentiation of syndromes. This differentiation is very difficult to see and requires the practitioner to be enlightened about the concept of "time."

Differentiation of syndromes is not similar to differentiation of disease. For example, if the patient has a headache in the forehead, modern Chinese medicine teaches that it is a stomach problem, because the stomach meridian reaches to this area. This diagnosis does not require enlightenment. As Mao Zedong claimed about the simplicity of this deduction, "Every uneducated person can learn it and learn it fast."

The analysis of the same headache from the classical Chinese medicine perspective is taken much further. It is a stretch of time, and not just an organ or a meridian, and must be dealt with in this way. The effectiveness of Chinese medicine is not in the modernized and scientific differentiation of symptoms, but rather the differentiation of life syndromes of often opposing forces that we call Yin and Yang.

If you train your brain in such classical Chinese thinking, then how you treat infertility takes an entirely different shape. It is no longer the treatment of symptoms, such as blood deficiency, or even worse, Western medicine diagnoses like Polycystic Ovary Syndrome (PCOS), high Follicle Stimulating Hormone (FSH), or endometriosis, of which the cause is forever "unknown." It is rather about the practitioner's ability to ensure not only a pregnancy, but more importantly, enable the mother, the baby, and the baby's offspring for generations to fulfill their heavenly years. For this reason, the treatment of infertility with classical Chinese medicine is of such great importance: one pregnancy and birth affects the many that will come later.

Chinese medicine realizes the truth in staying healthy and the importance of health for our future generations. Studies are not necessary to convince our common sense. We naturally trust our common sense. Understanding time means understanding health. Understanding health means that future generations will thrive.

TIME AND TWENTY-FOUR QI

He who well understands heaven will know man's life. He who well understands the ancient times will know its modern day's implications. He who well understands Qi will know its significance for any living matter.

—*The Yellow Emperor*

Throughout this book we will learn about heaven, ancient methods, and Qi (prounouced "chi"). The more we know about these three, the more we will understand infertility and how to become fertile.

Qi, which we call "life force," is the invisible force that gives us life. Each Qi corresponds to a phase of the moon, and there are two phases per month. The first phase, one Qi long, extends during the time the moon is born until it grows full; the second phase begins with a full moon and progresses until the moon is gone.

The twenty-four Qi help us understand that everything under heaven follows these rules of life. They make the big Qi of heaven more accessible here on earth. We realize that this big Qi, including the sun, earth, and moon, as well as day and night and the four seasons, all move in a circular motion. The twenty-four

Qi also describe lifespan, helping to segment the beginning, growth, and decline and end phases.

The sun's movement determines the twenty-four Qi, or segments, of the year. For the study of Qi, we must take the ancients' perspective that the sun circulates around us. It shines at us from the left, top, and right and then it travels through a zone where we can't see it. When we face south, sunrise is to our left and sunset is to our right.

The moon waxes and wanes twelve times in a year, absorbing the sun's energy, and reflecting the sun's light. However, every month the sun is in a different angle toward the earth, and during the course of a year, the sun moves in two opposite directions, north and south, creating two halves of the year: a birth and growth half, and a decline and storage half.

EACH OF THE TWENTY-FOUR QI OCCUPIES A HALF MOON CYCLE. THE SAGES ATTRIBUTED NAMES TO THEIR FUNCTIONS:

1. Xia Zhi — summer extreme
2. Xiao Shu — slight heat
3. Da Shu — big heat
4. Li Qiu — fall begins
5. Chu Shu — heat enters
6. Bai Lu — white dew
7. Qiu Fen — fall's split
8. Han Lu — cold dew
9. Shuang Jiang — frost descends
10. Li Dong — winter begins
11. Xiao Xue — slight snow
12. Da Xue — heavy snow
13. Dong Zhi — winter extreme
14. Xiao Han — slight cold
15. Da Han — great cold
16. Li Chun — spring begins
17. Yu Shui — water rain
18. Jing Zhe — hibernation startles
19. Chun Fen — spring's split
20. Qing Ming — obvious clear
21. Gu Yu — grain rain
22. Li Xia — summer begins
23. Xiao Man — small fullness
24. Mang Zhong — grain fullness

In the spring and summer there is an increase in heat, while in the fall and winter there is a decrease of heat.

Two kinds of Qi (energy) govern our life, Ming and Xing. Ming, our original Yang, is energy which comes from our parents, determines the heavenly years we have to live. Xing is the Yang energy that comes to us from heaven and the sun and helps us live our lives to the fullest. All living matter, including animals, trees and rocks, has a Ming, or internal fire, as well as a Xing, or external source of fire. The Earth itself has two kinds of fire, one emanating from the sun, and the other from the planet's core. Xing and Ming cannot exist without each other. For any life form to take place, we need these two kinds of "fire."

The twenty-four Qi describe, first and foremost, the relationship of the sun to our earth. In the northern hemisphere, when the sun is at its most northwestern point, its angle to earth is almost perpendicular and the temperatures are at their warmest. The Yang energy from the sun hits the earth's surface in the most direct way, causing the absorption ability, or Yin aspect, of the earth to decrease. As a result, the heat stays above the ground surface. In autumn, when the sun is moving toward the south, its light is less intense, and hence the ability of earth's Yin to absorb the Yang energy is increased. The sun's Yang energy gradually goes underground.

In winter, when the sun's intensity is weakest, the Yin energy is the strongest, the sun's Yang penetrating deep into the earth to warm what the sages called "the underground water." Going into spring, the sun travels back north, resulting in the Yin's decreased ability to absorb and the Yang's gradual reemergence onto the earth's surface, life springing out. As the sun reaches the north point, the summer is at full bloom again.

During winter and nighttime, the Yang energy goes into extreme storage inside the earth. This storage allows the Ming fire in the center core of the earth to survive. It also allows the Ming fire in the center of human beings to survive as well. The sun on the surface gives life, but the sun under the surface gives life too, just in a different way.

THE TWENTY-FOUR QI

1. XIA ZHI (summer extreme) – The sun arrives at the most northern point, or summer solstice. The weather is hot.
2. XIAO SHU (slight heat) – The first half of the moon following the arrival of the summer extreme, thus the heat above earth's surface is aggravating.
3. DA SHU (big heat) – The second half of the moon following the summer extreme. Heat above the surface is at its most extreme. The sages explaining Yin and Yang noted that the heat must arrive at its most extreme before reversing into cooling mode.
4. LI QIU (autumn begins) – The sun moves southward. Yang energy begins its descent toward earth.
5. CHU SHU (heat enters) – Yang energy first penetrates the earth's surface.
6. BAI LU (white dew) – Yang energy partially penetrates earth's surface, although more heat is still above the earth's surface than below it. Dew descends in early morning and possibly in late evening.
7. QIU FEN (fall's split) – Equal distribution of heat above ground and underground.
8. HAN LU (cold dew) – The heat underground more intense than the heat above ground. The Yin is now strong enough to pull most of Yang's energy underground. Temperatures above ground are cold; the morning dew feels cold to the touch.
9. SHUANG JIANG (frost descends) – Yin intensifies, most of Yang now under earth's surface. The morning dew freezes into frost.

10. Lɪ Dᴏɴɢ (winter begins) – The Yang sinks into the underground water or center core of the earth.

11. Xɪᴀᴏ Xᴜᴇ (slight snow) – The water begins to melt underground as more and more Yang and heat enter. Water above ground descends upon earth with no Yang, as snow.

12. Dᴀ Xᴜᴇ (heavy snow) – An increase in momentum from the previous step. The Yang is completely sunken into the underground water and the core of the earth. The underground water is the melted lava and hot springs coming from the center of the earth. The sun's Yang is supporting Ming.

13. Dᴏɴɢ Zʜɪ (winter extreme) – Arrival of the sun to its southernmost point.

14. Xɪᴀᴏ Hᴀɴ (slight cold) – The first half of the moon following the arrival of the sun in the south. The Yang is stuck inside and doesn't want to come out. The temperatures above ground are freezing cold.

15. Dᴀ Hᴀɴ (great cold) – The second half of the moon follows the sun's arrival in the south. The Yang storage underground reaches its extreme, while the temperatures above ground reach their extreme freezing point.

16. Lɪ Cʜᴜɴ (spring begins) – As the sun increases its angle with the earth, the pull of the Yin decreases. The Yang energy gradually exits the underground water, beginning its rising motion onto the earth's surface. Temperatures above ground warm up slightly.

17. Yᴜ Sʜᴜɪ (water rain) – Yang reaches the surface, rivers and lakes thaw and flow again.

18. JING ZHE (hibernation startles) – Yang is still more underground than above ground startling the hibernating insects underground, signaling the plants, insects, animals, and humans that the spring is about to take full force and it is time to come out.

19. CHUN FEN (spring's split) – The Yang energy is equally distributed above and below ground.

20. QING MING (obvious clear) – Most Yang is above ground, the temperatures warm and the leaves grow back on the trees. It is called "obvious clear" because we can see the full bloom of spring with our naked eyes.

21. GU YU (grain rain) – The Yang energy is completely above the ground's surface. The Yin forces are completely diminished. Due to sufficient Yang, the grains begin to grow. Enough Yang in the above ground water is called "rain." No Yang in the same water is called snow. Rain and snow signify the different position of the Yang above or underground.

22. LI XIA (summer begins) – The temperatures above ground are turning hot, as there is no Yin. The Yang floats above the earth's surface.

23. XIAO MAN (small fullness) – The grains on the ear begin to fill up. The temperature above ground is even hotter and the fruits and grains begin the process of ripening.

24. MANG ZHONG (grain fullness) – The Yang energy above ground is enough to cause grains and fruits to ripen, flavors at their climax.

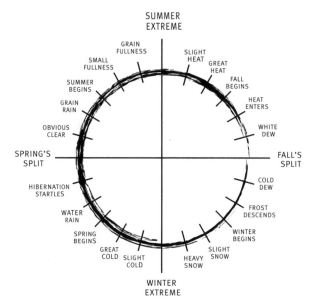

SUMMER
EXTREME

The sun's Yang is now floating above the surface and supporting Xing. It then moves back into position 1, the summer extreme. This is called the circular motion of the heaven's big Qi.

TWENTY-FOUR QI, HEALTH, AND FERTILITY

After we wake up from a good night's sleep, we feel stronger and recharged. The same is true of the Yang energy when it disappears from our sight during the night, and during the fall and winter. In both instances the visible sun and Yang go underground. The ancients saw the sun, and Yang, as performing a nourishing "keeping life" mission.

When the sun travels to the south and Yang energy enters underground in fall and winter, the life force is considerably nurtured, allowing a rebirth and a flourishing during spring and summer. From the perspective of the sages of Chinese medicine, nature has created these rules in order to preserve its own life.

Of the eighty-one chapters in *The Yellow Emperor*, the second chapter, "The Great Treatise of Harmonizing the Four Seasons with Qi and Spirit," is extraordinarily significant. Spirit in this context is a human being or a living entity on earth. The spirit is coming from heaven down into the living entity.

"The Yin and Yang of the four seasons are the root and foundation of the myriad things. Because it is the root, the sage nurtured the Yang in the spring and summer and he nurtured the Yin in the fall and winter. He followed the root of life so he could join the realm of birth and growth of the myriad things. If he would resist this root he will punish his own foundation and damage his own 'Truth.' Thus the four seasons and Yin and Yang are the beginning and end of the myriad things. They are the foundation of life and death. If you resist it, disaster will come, but if you follow it, disease will never rise. This is called Dao."

Harmonizing the four seasons and the twenty-four Qi with our spirit and with our life is crucial for our survival, health, and fertility.

For the enlightened sage of old, there was no need for medicine. He knew how to adjust his own rhythm to the rhythm of the four seasons and the Qi, thus preventing any and all diseases from taking hold of his body. Therefore, when we harmonize with the twenty-four Qi and the four seasons as the old sages did, it is the same. No disease can arise, including infertility.

Although we talk today about preventative medicine, nevertheless, we have no clue as to the root of life. We follow patterns of convenience under the false pretense that our life is an isolated unit, and that we can remedy it irrespective of nature, the four seasons, or the twenty-four Qi. This is why illness often overtakes us, even though we eat "right," pop supplements, and turn to promising drugs.

We are supposed to be impressed that today's life span is near eighty, up from forty-five at the turn of the twentieth century. However, 2,000 years ago, with no use of drugs, life expectancy for those who followed the Dao was one hundred. The root of our life is within the circular motion of nature. If we truly understand this notion, we can bring ourselves to the state of being where "disease will never rise," and where women will maintain their fertility until the age of forty-nine.

The second chapter of *The Yellow Emperor* continues by explaining how to follow the Dao in a practical way. We are urged to nurture the Yang in the spring and summer and nurture the Yin in the fall and winter. When we nurture Yin and Yang we can reach harmony with the four seasons. The tool we need to accomplish this task is the twenty-four Qi, which tells us how to harmonize with the four seasons at any point in time. *The Yellow Emperor* describes the different state of affairs in each season. In spring, the Yang gives birth to flowers and plants. In the summer, the Yang hovers above the surface, the tops of the trees full of life. Rarely do we look at the bottom of the tree trunk. In the autumn, however, when the leaves fall, we look downward at the earth's surface. The pulling down action of the earth is manifesting, the Yang "agitated."

The surface is where the exchange of heaven and earth occurs. It is the axis point between energies, or the Qi Jiao (Energy Exchange).

To understand this "agitation" of Yang in fall, we must compare the winter to the summer. The Emperor says that in summer, when the Yang is high above ground, the tops of the trees blossoming, the Yang is fully consumed. The sages called this glorifying of the exterior and diminishing of the interior. When the exterior flourishes, the interior dwindles. Thus the Yang in the fall becomes agitated, desperate to go back home to winter where it can sleep undisturbed while it recharges. If it doesn't come down, it will die.

The Emperor then goes on to explain the optimal sleep habits we need to adopt in order to harmonize with the four seasons. In the spring and summer, we should nourish the Yang by going to bed after dark and rising before dawn. In the fall and winter, we need to nourish the Yin by going to bed early. The same occurs in the fall where we wake up early as well, but in the winter we should rise after dawn.

In spring and summer, when the Yang is above ground, we must help it accomplish its task. We should go to bed late and wake up very early. This harmonizes our body with the Yang opening movement around us. It is often difficult to fall asleep in hot weather. When we use air-conditioning, we fall asleep earlier, because it is re-creating this condition of winter. However, any artificial re-creation of natural environments is risky, the Emperor warns, because the sage followed the root of life so he could join the realm of birth and growth of the myriad things. If he resists this root, he will punish his own foundation and damage his own "Truth." Faking winter in the middle of summer is resisting the root.

The character Zhen, which means "truth," is used to describe a

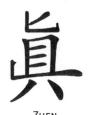

ZHEN

human being. It also translates to "a newcomer among the immortals." The Emperor warns that if you resist this root then you will not only harm your foundation (meaning your life), you will also harm your immortal life (meaning all your future generations).

This kind of long-term vision and wisdom is practically nonexistent in our modern world. The most we usually think about is one generation down to our children.

The Yellow Emperor describes some of the daily actions needed to harmonize with nature:

SPRING: Nourish the "Yang" by engaging in physical exercise, encouraging the stored energy below ground to emerge onto the surface of our body.

SUMMER: Because the Yang energy is above ground, we stay outside. We cannot get enough sun—we are insatiable. Any outdoor activity will cause our Yang to float to the surface and thus be synchronized with nature.

AUTUMN: We act as a rooster, bursting with energy in the morning but retiring early in the afternoon. Full vigorous physical activity should be done early in the morning.

WINTER: We must pattern ourselves after the sunlight, sleeping more to restore our energy and limiting physical activity.

The Yellow Emperor uses the word "must" in winter because the storage of Yang in this season has to do with our life expectancy, or Ming. In the other three seasons the wrong actions will impact our daily energy, or Xing. We may become ill, lethargic, or unproductive, but the impact on our life span will be minimal. In winter, if we do not act in the way that we must, and instead follow our heart's desires, then our Ming—our lifespan—will be shortened.

Thus the sage realized the importance of following sunlight in winter. He was to sleep longer hours during the winter, and also to keep physical activity to a minimum because the warming effects of the sunlight in winter are minimal. He was to be like the winter sunlight—mellow and subdued. His physical movements were to be slower and more contained.

In each season, we interact with a different state of energy, which means that in each season we must have a different state of mind. Maintaining the correct mindset is just as important as maintaining a physical regimen.

In spring, our intentions and ambitions rise. We interact more with nature and society. In summer, our ambitions are in the extreme. We project outwards, admiring our surroundings, interacting with them. In fall, the energy returns downward to the earth's surface, and our ambitions retract. We harmonize with nature by calming our spirit, drawing it back into our body. In winter, our ambitions and desires are withdrawn into a place where they are well hidden.

Of course, all of this stands in sharp contrast to our modern life, where we are constantly striving and never withdrawing or resting. We have lost our rhythm with nature.

When an infertility patient turns to storage and withdrawal during the winter, the chances of achieving conception in spring are greatly increased. This is called the Dao of nourishing "storage." When one reflects the spring in this way, it is referred to as the Dao of nourishing "birth." When one reflects the summer in this way, it is called the Dao of nourishing "growth." When one reflects the fall in this way, it is called the Dao of nourishing "gather."

If we don't allow our body and mind to follow the energy transformations in each season, there are consequences. If spring is resisted, the liver will be harmed, and as a result, the summer is cold and growth will be scarce. If summer is resisted, the heart will be harmed, and as a result the autumn "gather" energy will decrease and one will suffer fever and chills. Additionally, if summer is not followed, one will become severely ill in winter. If one resists autumn, the lungs will be harmed, and in winter storage will be scarce. If winter is resisted, the kidneys will be harmed, resulting in impotence and faint in the spring when "birth" will be scarce.

Let's focus on the winter and summer. *The Yellow Emperor* says that if summer is resisted, we will not only suffer "fever and chills" in the fall, we will become severely ill in winter.

Although *The Yellow Emperor* chooses summer's disharmony as a potential cause for a severe illness in winter, the truth is that resisting any of the three seasons will cause a severe illness in winter. And severe illness in winter means that there will be no ability to reproduce in spring.

As mentioned previously, our modern climate-controlled environments can make it difficult to be in tune with nature. If we heat up our homes in midwinter, we are not creating summer, we are creating an artificial summer. We are heating our home with oil, gas, or coal, all of which are extracted from the depths of the earth, which *The Yellow Emperor* refers to as "underground water." Because our artificial summer is derived from storage, the more storage we use in winter, the less we have to give birth in the spring.

Yet, *The Yellow Emperor* tells us that in winter we must expel the cold, then naturally it is warm; do not allow Qi to leak from the skin, bring the Qi urgently into containment. We cannot sweat because if we do, we will disconnect with nature and suffer impotence and faint in the spring.

From the perspective of the Classical Chinese medicine, leading a "healthy lifestyle" does not mean going to the gym or eating a "healthy" granola bar. It means that we need to understand nature. Since we are part of nature and not independent entities as modern society may lead us to believe, we must harmonize with it. If we do so, we will fulfill our heavenly years, and women will have the ability to become pregnant until the age of forty-nine.

SEPARATION VS. UNIFICATION

Our modern concept of time is linear. Today is today and tomorrow is tomorrow. Today and tomorrow cannot be the same thing. It is what we've learned since childhood as separation and differentiation. We, as Westerners, believe that when we separate and differentiate, we can tell right from wrong and good from bad.

In Chinese history and culture, the main driving factor is unification and harmony. Instead of saying "this is good and this is bad, let's avoid the bad," the Chinese ancients asked, "This is good and this is bad. How can we harmonize them together and make them work?" Instead of differentiating between today and tomorrow, the ancient sages tried to unify today and tomorrow. They tried to unify this year and next year. They were looking for the similarity in patterns instead of the difference. Or at least they were looking for the similarity in patterns so they could understand the difference between them.

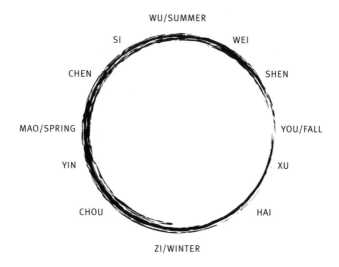

THE CHANGES SYSTEM

Energy-changing is the root of life. It is why we are on this planet, why we have plants and animals, oceans and land masses. The ancients realized that change, or Yi, is what makes the difference between life and death. But what is changing and how?

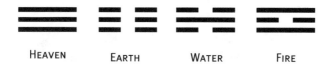

HEAVEN   EARTH   WATER   FIRE

Because these questions are difficult to answer, the Chinese sages developed the Yi, or "changes," system as something of an addendum to the Chinese characters. It is a system of images called trigrams, or "Gua," which are composed of three lines: either solid lines or broken lines. Solid lines represent Yang energy, while broken lines represent Yin energy.

By describing Heaven and Earth with the trigrams, the sages set the foundations for Chinese medicine development. "Heaven" is described with three solid lines, meaning that heaven is a pure

Yang energy phenomenon, with no Yin energy involved. Earth, on the other hand, is described with three broken lines. This indicates that earth is a pure Yin phenomenon.

To describe the "Yi," a before and after state are referenced, "Xian Tian," or Pre-heaven, and "Hou Tian," or Post-heaven. The "before" is before there was life, and the "after" is after there was life on earth. To understand life, health, and fertility we need to understand what happened in this change.

The Chinese classics describe life as an interaction between heaven and earth, or an interaction between Yang and Yin. If there is no interaction between heaven and earth, or no interaction between Yang and Yin, there is no life.

The ancients considered water and fire to be the basis for all life on earth because both are essential. For life to be created, the Yin and Yang must be in relationship, and to do this they must exchange their essence.

The ancients described the importance of water and fire to our lives in more than one way. They created a sequence of eight trigrams to portray the pre-heaven state and a different sequence of the same eight trigrams to portray the post-heaven state. (See illustration)

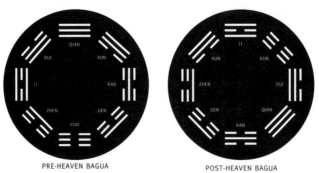

PRE-HEAVEN BAGUA   POST-HEAVEN BAGUA

This explains the different relationships of the trigrams before and after life was created. We can see in the pre-heaven trigrams that the positions of north and south are occupied by heaven and

earth. After the trigrams have changed to the post-heaven condition, these north and south positions are occupied by water and
fire respectively. This exchange explains that in prelife, heaven and
earth are pure Yin and pure Yang, and after life is created, they
must be water and fire.

Heaven and earth means the entire universe and all the life that
is in it. When the Yang essence is exchanged with the Yin essence,
water and fire are created, and therefore life is created. This is
exactly what happens between husband and wife in conception.

THREE YIN AND THREE YANG

The key to healing is to understand Yin and Yang. The most significant breakthrough of the sages in the Yin and Yang arena was the
dividing of the Yin and the Yang into six spheres, or segments—
three segments of Yang and three segments of Yin:

TAI YANG (great Yang)
YANG MING (bright Yang)
SHAO YANG (lesser Yang)

TAI YIN (great Yin)
SHAO YIN (lesser Yin)
JUE YIN (extinct Yin)

To understand three Yin and three Yang we have to go back to
nature, where the most pronounced Yin and Yang cycle is that of
the seasons. In the following illustration, please note that "south"
is at the top because in Chinese culture and history, all maps
display south at the top.

The spring belongs to the east and the fall belongs to the
west. The east is where the sun rises and that is where the energy
rises. The east energy is like the spring energy, where the plants

are springing upward and the energy is rising. The west is where the sun sets and the energy descends. The energy of the fall is descending when the leaves are falling back to the ground.

The energy of the universe has four stages. Spring is about birth, summer about openness and growth, fall about retraction, and winter about storage.

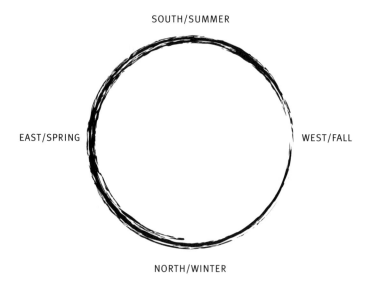

SOUTH/SUMMER

EAST/SPRING

WEST/FALL

NORTH/WINTER

In the past 500 to 700 years, some Chinese medicine practitioners with limited understanding of the ancient ways, and therefore limited understanding into the depth of Yin and Yang, began to categorize the four seasons in a logical way that distorted the course of Chinese medicine history. They claimed that because spring and summer are about opening up, they represent the Yang energy in nature, while fall and winter represent the Yin energy because they are about retracting and storing. This divided Yin and Yang into two halves, the feminine and the masculine. As Western philosophies were introduced into China about 400 years ago, this concept became even more widespread. Today, this idea is taught in acupuncture schools worldwide as the root of Chinese medicine. However, after much research of classic Chinese medicine the Yin and Yang should be understood on a deeper level in order for treatment to be more effective.

OPEN, CLOSE, AND PIVOT

The mechanisms behind these six spheres that make the Yin and Yang energies work are "opening," "closing," and "pivot." These movements act in succession, and together guarantee that life will go on without interruption.

The pivot is where the opening and closing actually takes place. It transforms the action of the energy, motivating the transition of the seasons. A door can be used as a metaphor. It needs a hinge to transform the static state of an unmovable slab of wood into a dynamic state of opening and closing. It transforms the door from a pre-heaven state into a post-heaven state. The two pivots are "Shao Yang" and "Shao Yin."

THE TAI YANG PHASE

The Tai Yang phase is the first phase of the energy transformation and is referred to as the birth of Yang energy. Tai Yang has several meanings in the Chinese language. It is called "Greater Yang" and is also the Chinese name for the sun, as well as for dawn as seen from the top of a mountain. It is the representation of birth and the representation of life. As long as there is expansion of energy, it is a time of "Tai Yang."

Understanding physical matter is a much simpler process than understanding the energies in the process of life. Physical process can be examined and observed under a microscope. With energy, or at least life-force energy, comprehension requires a depth of thinking. The deeper the thought, the more life is understood. When you understand life, you understand illness and are able to restore health. You are able to understand infertility and restore fertility.

In this process of gaining depth, we will describe the Tai Yang from different angles, therefore understanding it in a variety of ways.

The first angle is the birth concept. It is where the Yang (or great Yang or Tai Yang) is first born at midnight, or the time of Zi, in the middle of winter or when there is no moon. It stretches until Wu, which is noon or the middle of summer or full moon. It represents the time stretching from the moment we are conceived to our adulthood or midyears. In other words, it is the first half of all life as we know it, which is why Zhang Zhongjing dedicates half of his life work to Tai Yang.

The best exercise to deepen your understanding is to observe nature and its phenomena. The sun rises and sets, the moon waxes and wanes, the seasons change from warm to hot to cool to cold. When one contemplates these phenomena he can finally realize the repetitiveness of things and the regularity in them. The regularity in nature determines the rules by which we must abide. If we do, then health prospers and if we don't, then sickness follows. The exercise is to watch nature with the naked eye and write down in a notebook your findings, for example, "today is a full moon" or "today is a declining moon" and when your notebook is full with notes you compare the notes of one day to the other, one month to the other and find the repetitiveness or rules. This allows deepness of thinking.

The second angle to take in understanding Tai Yang is to look at its energy qualities. *The Yellow Emperor* describes these as "cold" and as "water."

Without water there is no life. What is the relationship between water, cold, and the Tai Yang? Tai Yang is the opening up of energy. What happens to water when the energy opens up or warms up? It evaporates skyward, or heavenward, where the cold atmosphere (cold energy) forces it back down to earth in the form of rain. When *The Yellow Emperor* describes Tai Yang as cold and water, he is referring to this phenomenon of water circulation that allows life on earth.

The third path to take in understanding Tai Yang is to relate it to the two organs that compose the Tai Yang sphere in the body—the bladder and small intestines. These two organs in the Chinese medical system are responsible for water metabolism. The small intestines digest the water, and the bladder controls the excretion of excess water. If the water metabolism is impaired, it is mainly because the Tai Yang system has a problem.

An impaired water metabolism affects our fertility. Part of the Tai Yang phenomenon is to help the water be distributed throughout the body in a proper and adequate way, areas with too much water sent to areas in need.

This stands in contrast to today's understanding of drinking and hydration. The trend today is to drink as much as possible in order to keep hydrated. When we constantly drink water, however, the Tai Yang organs are engaged in an excessive fashion. The bladder and small intestine are under extreme stress. On the other hand, some people don't have time to drink even if they are thirsty, which will cause a different set of problems. For normal Tai Yang water metabolism, we should strive for balance in drinking water. There is no such thing as one size fits all so each individual must find her own balance.

The fourth way to understand Tai Yang is to study the two meridians that compose the Tai Yang sphere: the bladder meridian, which is the most important, and the small intestine meridian. The bladder meridian starts at the inner cantus of the eye, runs along the top of the head and down the center of the back along both sides of the spine. It continues to flow down the posterior side of both legs until it reaches the lateral side of both little toes. It is the longest meridian, and the only one out of the twelve that is distributed exclusively on the posterior (back) side of our body.

When the Tai Yang is obstructed, the Yang energy cannot open up. If the Yang energy is only partially present when spring arrives, the flowers will seem poor and tired. It would be the same for people if the Yang energy did not open far enough when we wake up in the morning. We would feel lethargic and tired.

Because Tai Yang represents the sun, a warming force and source of light, we find it more difficult to wake up in colder weather. This is why *The Yellow Emperor* recommends less sleep in the summer. When the body encounters a burst of cold energy, such as when walking into a very cold air-conditioned office in the middle of summer, the opening of the Yang is obstructed. This can result in chills or catching a cold. We may experience a headache or stiff neck because the bladder meridian, running along the neck and head, is obstructed. We feel chills because the Yang energy can't open up to warm the body.

To remedy this obstruction, we must use warm herbs, such as cinnamon and Ma Huang (ephedra). These herbs can be ingested until minor perspiration appears. In other words, the best way to recover from a cold is to help the Yang expand, but to stop before sweating begins.

When and if you catch a cold stay away from drugs, use only herbs, chicken soup and rest as remedy, the body will take care of the rest. Stay away from cold places like an air-conditioned office or car, keep comfortably warm, not comfortably cold.

The Yellow Emperor notes that the Tai Yang enters and exits the body through the center of the chest. When we take Western medication for the common cold, many people experience the cold moving into the chest and then turning into a lingering cough. This is because we have not solved the obstruction of the Yang mechanism, we have simply pushed it a layer deeper. The entry and exit mechanisms have been obstructed. Using cold herbs to treat the common cold causes the same results.

If warm herbs are not used, then ingesting a hot rice soup and lying under blankets to rest should clear out the cold within a day or two. If you do not rest, keep warm, and drink warm soups, then the cold will move into the chest, obstructing the Yang and developing into a far worse situation such as a sinus infection. It will then be difficult to avoid Western drugs. Every action that we do to help preserve the Yang will help.

The Shao Yin is where all fertility happens. When the Tai Yang is obstructed, the Shao Yin suffers the consequences. In today's modern medicine of separating and differentiating one disease from another, the common cold is completely inconsequential to fertility. In Chinese medicine of unification and harmony, when the Yang mechanism is obstructed, the Shao Yin and fertility will suffer. Problems with the Yang mechanism are of course not only a consequence of the common cold but also of a variety of factors and situations that impact the Tai Yang channel. If this channel is kept open, the chances for fertility will greatly appreciate.

It is important to avoid overstimulation of the Tai Yang. Although it may feel like we are stimulating the Yang energy when we go to a party and stay out late, this can lead to exhausting the energy. The extra stimulation that we all experience from work, TV, or driving a car, as well as exposure to cold foods and cold drugs, causes our Yang energy to become more deficient.

To achieve fertility, it is important to begin modifying behavior and customs. For example, when you want an iced drink, try and do without it.

> To my patients I say, "it is time to get aggressive." In Chinese medicine, aggressive does not mean harsh drugs and surgeries, but rather do whatever it takes to become healthy, which includes changing your diet to nutrient dense food, changing your residence to a peaceful setting, quiet and full of fresh air, surrounded by trees, and change your job to a less stressful one. Get aggressive with everything around you in your lifestyle; however, never get aggressive with your own body.

A fifth aspect of the Tai Yang is the time when the energy is best open to a remedy for any imbalance. With Tai Yang, it includes the three months of summer on the lunar calendar, as well as 9 A.M. until 3 P.M., when the Yang energy is at its most open state.

THE YANG MING PHASE

The Yang Ming phase is the part of the Yang mechanism responsible for the closing down of the energy. It prevents the Yang from staying open forever. It has a protective action in preserving the Yang, ensuring its retraction into a storage phase. Farmers are well aware of the fact that if the winter is warm, the growing season the following year will be poor. Not sleeping well or long enough at night causes our energy level to be weak the following day.

The Yang Ming sphere occupies the time from Wu until Zi, or from noon until midnight, and from the midsummer, when the Yang energy is at its most open, until the midwinter, when it is completely stored. It is the part of our life from adulthood to death.

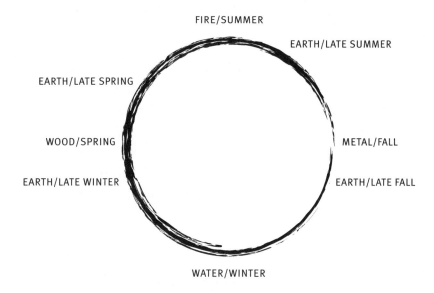

FIRE/SUMMER

EARTH/LATE SUMMER

EARTH/LATE SPRING

WOOD/SPRING

METAL/FALL

EARTH/LATE WINTER

EARTH/LATE FALL

WATER/WINTER

The third concept of Yang Ming is in relation to the organs of the body, specifically the stomach and large intestines, two organs that break down and expel the food we eat. These are both downward actions. The food's energy and nutrients come from heaven. We extract all the Yang energy from what we eat and drink so our life can continue. We allow all the turbid Yin and substance of the food to descend and be expelled as feces.

The fourth angle to take when approaching Yang Ming is its meridians. The large intestine meridian, which starts at the index finger, runs along the medial side of the arm and reaches the face from both sides at the nose. The stomach meridian, which starts at the face, runs downward along the front of the body until it reaches the tip of the second toe.

The Yang Ming meridians cover the entire front, or anterior, side of our body. Between the Tai Yang and Yang Ming, all of the Yang energy circulates up the back and down the front of the body. If both channels are working properly, we will feel energized and vital, and our health will be maintained.

When the Yang Ming becomes obstructed, the stomach and large intestines are full, which leads to possible constipation. The obstruction can occur from eating oily, greasy food that creates local heat. It can also be created by unnatural foods, such as modern processed food, artificial sweeteners, coloring, preservatives, or soft drinks. Common symptoms associated with constipation are shortness of breath, as well as insomnia due to the Yang's inability to go into storage at night. When the body can expel all unnecessary materials, a healthy state of Yang energy can be maintained. If the Yang cannot go into storage at night, it will bring on difficulty in sleeping.

With an apparent or local dryness, the bowels become dry and constipated. The symptoms associated with this pattern are heavy perspiration, a rise in temperature, a red face, and an intense, surging pulse. Heavy perspiration is the result of the body fluids evaporating out of the body like the wet laundry in the dryer. Feeling hot, as well as having a red face and an overactive pulse, are all signs of too much heat or the inability of the Yang to cool down. This will cause the Yang Ming to become dry and constipated, obstructing the Yang Ming downward cooling movement.

The Yellow Emperor suggests that the Yang Ming should be remedied from its center, which is Tai Yin "Damp" and "Earth." We should use moistening or dampness, or clearing the heat with the use of purgatives and cold herbs. As soon as the bowels restore their function, purgatives must immediately be stopped. This is because purgative and cold herbs damage the Yang energy, and with that, the life force. It is only a temporary localized heat that needs to be cleared so the Yang Ming can descend.

It should be noted that not all constipation is a Yang Ming issue, and other forms of the condition are not accompanied by perspiration, hot feelings, or having a red face. In ancient China, one could only use purgatives if it was a Yang Ming-related problem and only for a short period of time. If it was a Yang deficiency constipation issue, the Yang energy has to be strengthened, not purged.

With regard to the insomnia symptom associated with the Yang Ming obstruction, sleep medication will not solve the problem as it deals solely with the symptom and not with the cause. Instead of the Yang energy closing down, it is scattered. What may seem like a peaceful sleep is a completely different state of energy. When insomnia is caused by a Yang Ming obstruction, removing this obstruction will bring on sleep.

THE SHAO YANG PHASE

Shao Yang is described metaphorically by the Yellow Emperor as a pivot. It is the door hinge that allows the opening and closing of the Yang energy. We can see the Yang energy expression in its different phases of birth, growth, retraction and storage—the growth of the plants coming out of the earth, the leaves budding from the tree branches—but we cannot see the energy itself. It is like the seed of a plant, so small that if we drop it to the ground, we may not be able to find it again, but if we stick it in the ground, it may sprout a huge tree. The energy and potency is invisible like the Yang, yet it is there.

The energy without the seed, or without the Yin matter, will not work, nor will the seed without its energy. It is only when the seed and its energy are combined that we can get life. Shao Yang is the pivot that allows the Tai Yang and Yang Ming to continue and circulate. It is the force and quality that allows the Yang mechanism to repeatedly open and close without exhaustion.

The Shao Yang sphere ensures the continuation of life. It ensures that when we go to sleep at night, we will wake up in the morning to a new day, and when our Yang energy is consumed during the day, we will retreat to sleep to recharge. It ensures this life cycle of Yang energy will continue until we reach a point in our lives when it will be time to stop. It also has a crucial relationship with our fertility, which is what ensures a new generation, via its relationship with the Yin pivot, Shao Yin.

The second aspect of Shao Yang is its energy qualities.

Only when substance and energy meet—when earth and heaven meet—and exchange essence, is life formed.

It is the fire that warms up the body. It is the fire that gives us the appropriate energy to wake up in the morning and go to sleep at night. It is the energy that allows us to hear, see, smell, drink, eat, walk, run, write, read, talk, and laugh. It is the physical fire that makes us function.

The third aspect of Shao Yang is its organs, the gallbladder and the Triple Burner. In Chinese medicine anatomy, these two organs are in a very special, often misunderstood category. The Chinese medicine anatomy contains eleven organs—six Fu Yang organs and five Zang Yin organs. The Fu organs are hollow and allow movement of turbid matter to pass through. The stomach, small intestines, large intestines, bladder, triple burner, and gallbladder fall into this category. The five Zang organs store essence and do not allow movement through them. The heart, lungs, kidneys, liver, and spleen are in the Zang family. The gallbladder is in a special category because it stores bile and releases it for digestion. It has the function of a Yang organ and of a Yin organ simultaneously. It is called an extraordinary organ.

San Jiao, or the triple burner, is unique in that it is the only "organ" in the Chinese medicine anatomy which is not a physical organ, but is pure function. Containing three "burners" that transmit the minister life's fire throughout the entire body, it also provides the passageway for body fluids to be distributed. The upper burner includes the lungs, heart, and brain and is the root of our spirit. The lower burner includes the kidneys and liver and is the root of our essence and substance. The middle burner, the root of our post-heaven life, includes the spleen and stomach, and is where the food and liquid come into our body, giving us the life force or the fire we need.

The fourth aspect of Shao Yang is the triple burner meridian and gallbladder meridian. The triple burner meridian starts at the ring finger, travels upward through the center of the arm between the Tai Yang and Yang Ming channels, then runs along the side of the neck and the side of the head. The gallbladder meridian runs along the side of the head, down the side of the rib cage and side of the legs until reaching the fourth toe. When a person stands upright with arms relaxed at both sides of the body, both meridians run exactly on both sides of the body between the front, which is the Yang Ming channel, and the rear, the Tai Yang channel. The Shao Yang is the connecting factor between the two.

It is on the sides because Yin matter goes downwards and Yang energy goes upwards. This is the concept of the Shao Yang meridian distributed on both sides of the body.

The fifth aspect of Shao Yang is the time for unlocking, or remedying, which includes the times of Yin, Mao, and Chen. These times make up the daily cycle from 3 A.M. until 9 A.M., and represent the three months of spring in the Chinese lunar calendar. It is a time of "kindling warmth" as opposed to the summer's robust fire, very gentle warmth that spreads around in nature, causing plants to spring from the ground and birds to emerge.

The Yang energy of Shao Yang is a gentle fire that promotes growth and development. It is different than the pathological fire we have seen in the Yang Ming section that can cause dryness and constipation. It is the minister fire or the kindling warmth that is needed for our metabolism and it is achieved with the help of bile from our gallbladder.

The spring and the early morning hours possess this unique quality of light warmth. It is the energy in nature that promotes a healthy Shao Yang function, and is the reason Chinese medicine recommends consuming the day's main meal in the morning, a light meal at lunch and a small snack for dinner. The morning warmth is what aids the metabolism and digestion. Eating large dinners and small breakfasts will cause the Yang mechanism to suffer greatly, and is one reason why maintaining the wrong eating habits can cause disharmony, even with a healthy diet.

An imbalance in the Shao Yang may cause a bitter taste in the mouth, a dry throat, and blurry eyes. Bitter is the flavor of fire, dryness the pathology caused by fire, and blurriness the result of flaring fire or pathological fire. Shao Yang problems are caused by fire: not a minister's or "kindling wood" fire, which is just warm enough to help metabolism but is not too hot to obstruct it.

The main cause for Shao Yang obstruction is emotional stress. This is especially prevalent to infertility patients going modern ART treatment. The emotional anxiety hinders the pivot function of Shao Yang and disease may follow. Keeping the pivot unobstructed is done by unobstructing the emotions, which in turn is being accomplished by ridding oneself of stress factors, and this may include avoiding doctors who put you in despair. Avoiding emotional stress at home and at work is key.

Three organs are most prone to opening and closing: the mouth, throat, and eyes. The mouth opens and closes for Yang (talking) and for Yin (receiving and chewing food). The throat opens and closes for Yang (breathing) and for Yin (swallowing food, drinks, and saliva). The eyes open and close for Yang (to catch light and vision) and for Yin (to allow Yin storage and tears). If the pivot or the hinge is obstructed in any of these, the opening and closing will suffer. This will cause pathological heat or not enough warmth. If this happens, the body needs to harmonize.

Another main symptom of the Shao Yang disease is an alternating cold and hot feeling, frequently experienced after taking fertility drugs. Premenopause symptoms such as hot flashes can at times fall under this category as well. Other symptoms include pains along the sides of the body, or a headache on one side of the head, signaling an obstruction of the Shao Yang meridians, as well as decreased appetite and nausea due to a need for the spleen energy to ascend and the needs of the stomach's energy to descend. The Shao Yang minister fire needs to harmonize this upward and downward separation.

Energy disharmony can be brought about by emotions. Certainly, anxiety associated with the inability to conceive can have a negative effect on fertility.

Most body functions require harmonizing and need the Shao Yang's minister fire to help. This includes the reproductive organs of both women and men. Shao Yang's root is fire (minister fire), its manifestation is hot as it harmonizes the Yang energy, and its center is Jue Yin, which will be discussed in a later section and includes the liver organ, a major player in creating or preventing fertility and reproduction.

THE TAI YIN PHASE

When we reach the Tai Yin, or the Yin within Yin, we have reached the physical living organism. The Tai Yin is where physically living matter interacts with other physically living matter. For example, the living parts of food and drink (nutrients) interact with the Tai Yin spleen organ. Air that we breathe interacts with the Tai Yin lung organ. Water is the embodiment of the Yin state. It contains life because it has warmth, or Yang energy, within. The warmer the water, the more life there is. The Tai Yin anchors the Yang energy into the body. Without it, the Yang would float away.

The second aspect of Tai Yin is its energetic qualities, described by *The Yellow Emperor* as "Damp" and "Earth." Earth, described in earlier chapters, is the expression of solid matter. It symbolizes the body's tissues, such as the bones, flesh, skin, and inner organs. All living things spring from the earth, so it has additional meaning. Earth is closely related to water and dampness.

The third aspect of Tai Yin is its organs—the spleen and the

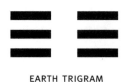

EARTH TRIGRAM

lungs. The spleen is responsible for receiving the Yang energy from food and drink. This is referred to as the root of the post-heaven energy—where we get our energy after we're born. When we choose the foods we eat, it is important to consider whether or not it contains Yang, or heaven energy. Natural food has heaven energy because it is produced by heaven and earth. When food is harvested, its natural instinct is to perish, because once it is removed from nature its Yin matter and Yang energy want to separate. Today's food industry processes and packages food so that it can stay on the shelf for months and even years. From a Tai Yin perspective, the recent trend toward consuming more locally grown fresh food is very wise.

The lungs, like the spleen, are responsible for the post-heaven energy received into our body after we are born, as opposed to the energy we receive from our mother while in the womb. The lungs are responsible for taking the heaven's Yang from the air and inserting it into our body as we breathe. Both Tai Yin organs receive the Yang energy in its different forms and then insert it into our body's physical matter. The reason this is important is because the Tai Yin sphere is responsible for anchoring the Yang energy into physical matter.

The fourth aspect of Tai Yin is its meridians: the spleen meridian and the lungs meridian. When a person stands upright with both hands to the sides of the body, the Tai Yin meridians are distributed along the inside of the arms and legs (medial side). Their location on the body facilitates the job of the meridians, which is to bring the condensed Yang energy into the body tissues. They bring the Yang within Yin or the Yang within the matter into the body.

The fifth aspect of Tai Yin is the unlocking times that represent the three months of winter in the lunar calendar, and in the daily cycle they are from 9 P.M. until 3 A.M. In order to understand this fifth aspect thoroughly, it is important to understand the three Yin spheres, which are more closely related than the Yang spheres, and often interchangeable. In addition, the three Yin meridians can be difficult to separate. This is because the Yin mechanism, while still opening, closing, and pivoting, occurs inside the Yin material.

The time of Hai (9 P.M.–11 P.M.) is when the Yin is pure and the Yang is in complete storage. The time of Zi, one hour before midnight, is where the first Yang—the Tai Yang—is born. The Yang then grows during the time of Chou (1 A.M.-3 A.M.). Sleep is important because when the Yang rises within the Yin, it is similar to the steam elevating from cooked rice. It provides life inside the house—life inside our body. It is important to sleep at the right time so the body becomes harmonious with nature.

When we have an obstruction of the Tai Yin sphere, sleep is a remedy. Symptoms associated with this obstruction generally begin with the abdomen–the center of the body that belongs to the earth—feeling full or bloated, signaling that the Yang is not transforming the Yin harmoniously. For example, when an infertility patient receives medication, the abrupt stimulation of Yang brings the Tai Yin into disharmony, often resulting in a bloated feeling. In Western medicine, this is referred to as a "side effect." In Chinese medicine, this phenomenon is a "disharmony." Pain in the abdomen is the result of cold, which signifies the absence of Yang—where the Yang energy does not transform the Yin substance and (Yin) energy and the Yin becomes obstructed.

In Chinese medicine, the time from 9:00 P.M. until midnight is when the body rejuvenates its blood (material). If we sleep at this time, our blood will be vigorous and many of our ailments solved, including fertility. The first thing that an infertility patient needs to consider is to change his or her sleeping patterns. Going to bed at 9:00 P.M. for several months will greatly increase the chance of conception.

In addition, allowing fresh air and the moonlight to enter the room is an advantage. Complete darkness doesn't allow the body to harmonize with the lunar rhythm.

In our daily lives, drinking cold drinks, eating cold foods, consuming cold herbs and cold medications lead to the obstruction of Tai Yin. Preserving the Yang energy of the spleen (Tai Yin) is the most important factor in the treatment of any disease.

THE SHAO YIN PHASE

Shao Yin is the pivot of the Yin mechanism, and is so closely related to the Tai Yin that they could be said to be inseparable. Water and earth, as well as water and fire, need the Yang energy in order to create life. The Shao Yin is the embodiment of this. The essence of the pure Yin (earth) and the pure Yang (heaven), the living Yin (water) and the living Yang (fire) is all within the Shao Yin. The interaction between heaven and earth in the body, and the way water and fire complement each other, are all functions of the Shao Yin, the Yin mechanism's pivot.

In Chinese medicine, a person's actions and events over a lifetime are all consequential to his or her Shao Yin sphere and reproductive ability. This includes longtime eating habits, sleeping habits, and the way in which ailments have been treated. It even includes how the individual's parents ate, slept, and treated ailments before they were born.

The second aspect of Shao Yin is its energetic qualities. *The Yellow Emperor* refers to the Shao Yin as "Emperor's fire." The Emperor Fire in our body is the sphere that unifies the body and emotions. In the body, the heart is like the emperor. It is the organ that allows this unity in the body. The reason for two kinds of fire in the six spheres is that the Shao Yang fire warms up the body, while the Shao Yin fire lights up the body. The emperor fire represents the brightness of the light.

The third aspect of Shao Yin is its organs, the kidneys and heart. The kidneys belong to the water element, while the heart belongs to the fire element. This represents the water and fire interaction within the body.

In the body, the heart is like the emperor. It is the organ that allows this unity in the body. The spirit in heaven and earth represents the energetic qualities of each of the six spheres. The Tai Yang sphere is cold and water, the Jue Yin sphere is wind and wood, the Yang Ming is dryness and metal. Tai Yin is earth and mist. Only Shao Yang and Shao Yin unite into one category where one is heat and one is fire, which are the two aspects of the same fire—heat and light. The spirit is the mechanism connecting us to heaven and earth. It is the mechanism and unifying factor that connects us to nature, allowing the Yang (heaven) and Yin (earth) to interact within our bodies.

When the Yin and Yang separate at death it is said that the spirit has departed. So what does it mean that the spirit is clear? Let us

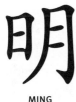

MING

look into the character Ming. The left side represents the sun, the right side represents the moon. These are the two most clearly lit objects in the sky.

The Yellow Emperor describes the heart as "the emperor where Shen Ming comes out." Loosely translated, it means that the heart is where the spirit becomes clear, and the spirit sees everything. The emperor fire is the light that is needed for the spirit to see what is happening in every part of the body. All ailments are caused by the spirit that is not clear because it is in the dark and cannot see.

Western medications such as pain relievers are actually a hindrance to solving the root problem of any physical issue because they remove the light from the spirit in order to relieve the symptoms. The emperor can no longer see what is happening in his kingdom. The same can be said for infertility procedures. If a patient who undergoes IVF treatments doesn't feel side effects such as hot flashes, weight gain, or abdominal distension and bleeding, it is because the spirit is now clouded and medication side effects are masked. Therefore, the spirit is not clear and the emperor fire is not shining the light that it should.

The heart organ is the most important organ and contains the most important function in the body. Without it, the body cannot see and repair ailments, connect to natural surroundings, or connect to heaven and earth. The body's Yin and Yang energies are in chaos. In Chinese medicine, the heart fire combined with the kidney Yang is called "True Yang."

Qiang has two meanings. It translates to "rice worm," which resembles a male's penis, and is the Emperor's way of describing the kidneys' control of the reproductive organs (male and female). The second meaning is strength. That "the kidneys are the officer of

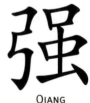

QIANG

Qiang" means that the kidneys, which belong to the water element, rule this quality of maintaining a hardness and softness simultaneously. This quality, however, cannot be separated from the heart.

The heart is where the spirit becomes clear and the kidneys control the hardness and softness of the genitalia. These are the preliminary conditions for reproduction. When the male and female become intimate, the emotions are even. If male stimulation or anxiety is too great or too little, or there is a lack of desire, the male will not experience erection. The same is true with female arousal. Too much and too little are both counterproductive. The heart is where the spirit resides and the emotions are kept in check. When the spirit is calm and the emotions content, or when there is love, the emperor fire can go down to the kidneys and warm up the kidneys' water. The kidneys' water will allow the Qiang to bend and straighten and reproduction to take place.

In contrast, IVF and timing ovulation, instead of warming the heart's emotions, is cooling the fire off. It separates the heart's fire from the kidney's water. And as the Yellow Emperor states, "The kidneys control hibernation. They are the root of storage. They are the place of essence." Hibernation is when we sleep and recharge our energy for the next day.

Preserving hibernation is when we sleep well. Preserving the essence is when we follow the guidelines of Shao Yin. We nourish the emperor's fire of the heart (emotions and clear state of mind) and keep the one true Yang of the kidneys.

Steroid use unleashes the true Yang in the kidneys, the body healing as if with a miracle. But the Yang is depleted—it is consumed. With hormone stimulation in fertility treatments, it is a similar situation in that the Yang in the kidneys becomes depleted. This depletion is antithetical to conception. As the Yellow Emperor said, "The Yin and Yang must harmonize. This will give birth to an offspring." If the Yang is depleted and can't be harmonized with the Yin, this will cause infertility.

The fourth aspect of Shao Yin is its meridians of the kidneys and heart. When one stands upright with hands to the side, palms touching thighs and the feet close together, the Shao Yin meridians run along the inside of the body on the posterior side (the inside of the arms and legs but close to the back). The inside of the body is Yin and the posterior part is Yang, thus it is the Yang within the Yin. The heart and kidney's meridians start in concealed areas under the feet and under the armpits, thus their origin is concealed in the pre-heaven. In other words, the Shao Yin energy comes from our parents, so we can't see its beginning.

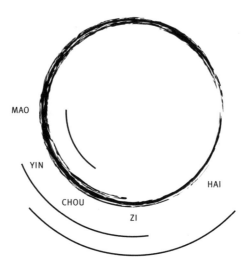

Shao Yin is the embodiment of heaven and earth interacting within the body. It is the kidney water and heart fire that act like the heaven and earth in nature. The Shao Yin, like the Shao Yang, is the pivot, and the pivot belongs to fire, the driving force behind the Yin and Yang. In the Yin mechanism, the fire is less warming than in the Yang mechanism, yet it is a full body of Yang within the Yin that drives the Yin mechanism into change. That is why the unlocking time of the Shao Yin is entirely within the Yang growth phase.

When the Shao Yin becomes obstructed, the pulse is thin and small, and the body wants to sleep but cannot. The heart feels irritable, urination is clear and frequent, and thirst is pronounced.

Additional symptoms of the Shao Yin imbalance include frequent urination of clear urine. This has to do with the Yang's failure to warm up the kidneys. When Yang is too intense, the kidneys warming up too much, the urine turns yellow, but when Yang is lacking, the urine is clear. There is no heat in the urine.

The most important symptom in the Shao Yin is the thin and small pulse, which is again a problem of water and fire. Fire is the energy and water is the substance. The most "water-like" substance in the body is blood, as it fills the veins and arteries. If the blood (water) is missing, the pulse will be thin. This is in contrast to a full-bodied pulse where the blood is ample. A small pulse is a fire problem, or to be more accurate, an emperor fire problem. How is it an emperor fire problem?

First, let's consider the minister fire that must warm the body. When there is too much warmth, the pulse turns rapid and when there is lack of warmth (or cold) the pulse turns slow. This is because warmth and Yang accelerate the water, while cold slows it down. The pulse within our body is the embodiment of life. The cycle of every heart beat in a pulse is similar to every day's cycle and every year's cycle. Each pulse has a spring, summer, fall, and winter. There is a cyclical and repetitive movement to it. The winter is the water or the blood of the pulse or the Yin energy of the pulse. The spring, summer, and fall are the Yang energy of the pulse.

In each heartbeat, a long spring, summer, and fall pulse should be felt. If the pulse is short it means that the Yang or emperor fire mechanism of the kidneys is in decline. It is the heart's spirit that harmonizes the seasons and the body. When a person's heart fire is healthy and the kidney's true Yang is strong, the pulse is long.

Infertility is to a large degree a Shao Yin problem. The emperor fire does not warm the kidney's true Yang. The spirit does not store in the essence. The energy does not root in the matter. The common symptoms that I encounter with most infertility patients are Shao Yin symptoms of Yang deficiency such as cold hands and feet, or a cold nose, while others feel hot flashes and night sweats. There is not enough warm (Yang) energy to warm you.

How can we understand hot flashes and night sweats as Yang deficiency? Straight symptoms are cold feet, cold hands, pale face, etc. There are, however, odd symptoms like red face and feeling hot. This is because the water contains the pre-heaven Yang. When the Yang is deficient, the water overflows and carries the original Yang with it upwards. The original Yang (emperor fire) should go downwards to warm the water; however, when it is deficient it cannot go downwards and floats upwards instead. This will give rise to symptoms such as hot flashes and night sweats. When the true Yang is strong again, the Yang will root into the water and will not float upwards.

In my practice, I recognize that hot flashes and night sweats of the Yang deficiency type can be alleviated rather quickly with very hot herbs. The worse the night sweats and hot flashes, the hotter the herbal formula needs to be. This is in order to save the Birthing Yang from separating. What is the main cause of infertility? The true Yang in the water is deficient and the emperor fire is too weak to descend.

In my experience, patients who have never used fertility drugs or birth control pills restore their true Yang and emperor fire rather quickly and easily. Patients who have used fertility drugs and birth control pills restore the water's true Yang with great difficulty.

Lack of true Yang explains why many IVF cycles fail, despite a successful embryo transfer. It also explains most "unexplained" infertility.

Restoring the Yang happens when one changes his/her lifestyle in such a way that brings harmony with nature. When one changes his behavior according to the seasons, for example, outgoing in summer and withdrawn in winter, sleeps according to the sun's movements, eats his food according to nature's rules, for example, unmodified food without pesticides, then the harmony with nature brings back the Yang. When we lose the harmony with nature on any level: diet, lifestyle, emotional or spiritual, we then waste our Yang.

THE JUE YIN PHASE

Jue Yin is the last sphere of the Yin mechanism. It is where Tai Yin and Shao Yin come to an end, enabling Yang to flourish. While Tai Yin is true Yin and Shao Yin is Yang within Yin, Jue Yin is Yin within Yang. The closing of Jue Yin finds itself entirely within the Yang realm.

When we compare the three Yin phases to fertility and reproduction, Tai Yin is the creation of the sperm and egg, Shao Yin is the conception and creation of a new life, and Jue Yin is the development of the fetus within the mother. Jue Yin is already a new life separated from the previous cycle (from the parents) yet it is still connected to the mother and not truly independent. It is only when the baby is born that the Jue Yin phase has completed its work and is an entirely independent new cycle.

The second aspect of Jue Yin is its energetic qualities. *The Yellow Emperor* describes Jue Yin as "Wind and Wood." The character of wind is composed of two parts.

The Chinese sages said, "the wind is the messenger of heaven and earth." This meant that all living things, humans included, are the messengers of heaven and earth. Human beings in particular were considered the mirror of heaven and earth interaction. They are the embodiment of Yin and Yang and life. Jue Yin, being the life already created but not yet separated from its parent, is best described by wind. What is the quality that describes this fetal phase so well? It is wood.

What is the connection between wind and wood? *The Yellow Emperor* says, "the east gives birth to wind and the wind gives birth to wood." The east, the wind, and the wood are three different layers of the same thing. The east is where the sun, or Yang energy, rises or comes out of the earth. This Yang energy gives birth to wind, which represents all living things on earth. The living things (wind) give birth to wood, to reproduction, and ultimately, to the next generation. Wind and wood cannot be separated. Life and reproduction cannot be separated.

Tai Yin and Shao Yin "come into extinction," as the Yellow Emperor says, by the birth of a new life, or by the wind giving birth to wood. Jue Yin is important to solving infertility because it allows us to understand miscarriages and the health of the fetus.

The third aspect of Jue Yin is its organs, the liver and the pericardium, a double-walled sac that contains the heart and the roots of the great vessels. The Yellow Emperor calls the pericardium "the walls surrounding the emperor (heart)."

When we think about the heart "sac" or pericardium, we are focusing on a fetus. When a baby is not yet born, it is inseparable from its mother. Jue Yin is the "extinction" of Yin into a new life, "extinction" in this instance meaning new birth.

The Yellow Emperor says: "When the Yin reaches its highest peak, the Yang is born." The cycle of Yin and Yang, or the cycle of life and birth, is happening all the time. It happens in a woman's life span when she gives birth to a child. It happens in a year's span, when winter gives birth to spring. It happens in the span of a day, when night gives birth to the morning, and it also happens within a heartbeat. When the heart beats once, it is a new life that was just born. It is a new push of blood and energy into our body. What happens when the heart stops beating? There is no birth; there is not another life in another beat, and no additional cycle of life. When we refer to the heart sac and the fetus in the sac, we mean the heart muscles pumping the blood and energy to allow us "life." It is a description of how our life is continuing. The pericardium is not a mere muscle like the muscles of the leg. It is the organ with which the spirit connects, where heaven and earth pump life into our body.

The Yellow Emperor further describes the Shan Zhong (center of the chest/pericardium) as the faithful minister, the one who obeys the emperor without deviation. It is the faithful blood pump that never fails us.

The Yellow Emperor analogizes the liver as the army general and defines it as the organ from which thinking and planning emerge. The liver functions are important for our life in the same way that an army general is important to the army. If the general thinks and plans strategically and thoroughly, his army will be victorious in a time of war.

A state of war exists when the Yin phase (storage) wants to transform into a Yang phase (expansion). In our daily life, a state of war exists every morning when we wake up, when sleep changes into waking. Yang energy wants to separate, but Yin energy wants things to stay together. This war between Yin's wishes and Yang's wishes is called Jue Yin. The liver is the general who has to plan how to win this war. If the liver fails in planning this transition, the war will be lost, and the body will not wake up. If the liver fails to plan, a baby will not be born. A pregnancy is a war over the baby's continued attachment to the mother or separating from her. If the liver function fails due to poor planning, and the baby separates too early, there will be a miscarriage. If the baby does not separate at term, a stillbirth will occur.

In Chinese history, the ultimate victory is to defeat the opponent before the war has even started. This is achieved with a well-planned strategy. In our daily life, a healthy liver delivers this well-planned strategy providing a seamless transition from Yin into Yang. If the liver is unhealthy the planning will be poor and a woman will have difficulty maintaining a pregnancy or having a healthy baby.

The Yellow Emperor states: "The liver harmonizes the tendons and ligaments, and its function is to straighten and bend." The liver is concerned with the flexibility we have in our body, especially in the joints. The liver function allows us to bend forward and sideways, and to stretch and bend our arms, hands, fingers, and knees. We previously mentioned the wood element and its function to "straighten and bend" as related to the male genetalia. A poor diet, inadequate sleep, excessive stress, or the taking of medication, will damage the liver. The army's general can no longer plan effectively. Pregnancy will be harmed.

The Yellow Emperor goes on to say that: "When a person lies down, the liver receives the blood and the person's eyesight is clear. When the feet receive the blood, he can walk." When the hands receive the blood, he can grasp. This refers to the all-important liver function of regulating the blood system, or life force, in the body. This is different from blood circulation, but rather the harmony of Yin and Yang.

When the life force—the correct combination of Yin and Yang energy—reaches any particular part of the body, this part will function, including the uterus, ovaries, and fallopian tubes. To achieve this harmony, we must first harmonize the liver.

The Yellow Emperor states that the liver receives the blood when the person is lying down; he is referring to the Wei position or the posture taken when a couple lies together to conceive a new life, or when a person goes to sleep trying to conceive a new life for the next day. The liver is receiving the life force when the person is creating a new life. The liver is the army general and should plan how this will happen; in order to do so, however, the eyes must be clear. When the energy goes into the liver for procreation, the vision must be clear for the sperm to know which egg to visit, and the egg to know which sperm to receive.

The Yellow Emperor goes on to state that "all channels (meridians and blood vessels) belong to the eyes." Many meridians go through or connect to the eyes; however, the eyes, able to tell good from bad, are related to all organs of the body. Any harm to the body (illness or injury) will make the eyes blurry, obstructing the liver's ability to harmonize Yin and Yang in order to create a new life. Pregnancy will be impossible to sustain. This is how the liver is related to the Jue Yin phase of creating a new life.

The fourth aspect of Jue Yin is the liver and pericardium meridians, running along the middle of the median side of our arms and legs. It is interesting to note that the liver meridian is circulating through the genitalia and the reproductive organs. Since one of Jue Yin's main functions is to allow a new life to develop, it makes perfect sense that Jue Yin meridian will nourish the reproductive organs. The liver meridian has internal pathways that circulate to the crown of the head, which is the most Yang area of our body. The meridians of Jue Yin also explain the connection of wind-wood and the minister fire, and how together, they create life. Without the warmth of the minister fire, the new life will not have Yang energy needed to evolve itself.

The Yellow Emperor explains by saying, "Yang energy is like the relationship of the sun to heaven. If the sun loses its place in the heaven, life will stop and the greatness of life is gone. So when the sky is turning, the sun must shine. This is the reason that Yang is above and protecting us from the outside."

This shows that even though Yin is crucial for life, Yang is the source of life. Waking up in the morning is Yang energy. Creating a baby from an egg and sperm is Yang energy. *The Yellow Emperor* says that Yang energy of our body is like the sun in the sky and is the reason why Yang is above, protecting us from the outside. The sun in the sky is crucial for life in the same way that Yang energy is crucial for life. Yang is defending us from ailments and is nourishing life.

It is important to preserve Yang energy. The sun will never stop shining, but our Yang can be finished because we belong to the earth. The energy in our material is borrowed from heaven. If we preserve Yang, we will live longer, healthier lives and be able to give this Yang "seed of life" to a new generation.

Harmony with nature is key. When a person beats in harmony with nature his heaven's given Yang is being spent less. It takes less energy to live and by default prolongs its existence. Yang existing for a long time means that our life exists for a long time. The sages of Chinese medicine understood that preserving Yang equals not wasting it. Being in harmony with the natural laws of nature keeps the Yang, while going against nature brings about its demise. Throughout the book I discuss desired actions that bring about harmony, and harmful actions that must be avoided. Follow the wisdom of the ancients in order to preserve your Yang.

What happens when Jue Yin becomes obstructed? Symptoms include thirst, hunger with no desire to eat, and vomiting when one does eat, as well as a hot and painful heart, meaning a heart attack. A patient who purges downwards with cold herbs will produce endless diarrhea.

But if we can keep our wind healthy and unobstructed, the body will solve all minor problems naturally. There will be no need for over-the-counter, under-the-counter or behind-the-counter medications.

Our Yang energy goal is to harmonize with the surrounding nature so Yin energy will not be affected. When Yang energy fails or becomes exhausted, Yin energy is impacted. The first line of Yin energy to be affected is the Tai Yin spleen, which is a simple problem. Strengthening the spleen will return the body to a healthy course. Beyond that, advancing pathology into Shao Yin and Jue Yin is very difficult and complicated, which normally happens with the elderly, where energy has been exhausted and the body's defenses are absent or low. Then, pathological progression into the core of life can be present. What I find alarming is that so many young people today have Shao Yin and Jue Yin syndromes — chronic diseases such as heart problems, diabetes, and cancer.

Most infertility patients are Tai Yin patients. Their bodies still work well at the core, yet something is missing which can easily be fixed. Other patients that I see, unfortunately, do belong to the Shao Yin–Jue Yin pattern of disharmony, generally due to the consumption of excessive Western medications. These compounds invade the core of life, or into what Chinese medicine calls "wind," and throw it into disharmony.

For thousands of years, while Chinese Philosophy has been about flowing with nature, the Western philosophy has been about conquering nature. Most Western medications are xxx-blocker or xxx-antagonist, and so on. They attempt to interfere with body functions in order to create a new scenario, which is not what nature intended.

THE FIVE ELEMENTS

The theory of the five elements is at least 2,500 years old and has set a foundation for understanding the universe and ourselves. Over the centuries, many physicians used it to perfect their healing skills. In the five elements, we can see the five species, five colors, five flavors, five emotions, five grains, and so on. They are part of the six heavenly energies, and are also present in the five earthly energies.

As stated previously, the five elements are wood, fire, earth, metal and water. There are two basic relationships between the elements: one is a generation relationship and the other a controlling one. Sheng, the generating relationship, describes the generation of one element from the other: the way wood gives birth to fire, fire gives birth to earth, earth gives birth to metal, metal gives birth to water and water gives birth to wood. It is a complete cycle of one element generating another over and over again.

With the second basic relationship Ke, the controlling relationship, the elements check each other to make certain they are in balance and not excessive. Wood controls earth, earth controls water, water controls fire, fire controls metal, and metal controls wood again. This cycle is endless.

There are, in addition, specific rules for the behavior of the elements: Sheng (overcontrolling), Cheng (adverse reaction) and Fu (revenge). These are abnormal actions of the elements defined by the Yellow Emperor.

When these control and generation cycles go out of balance, disease arises. For simplification purposes, let us refer to the elements as A, B, C, D, and E. A gives birth to B, B gives birth to C, C gives birth to D, D gives birth to E, and E gives birth to A. In the controlling cycle, A controls C, B controls D, C controls E, D controls A, and E controls B. When A, for example, is overcontrolling C, it is referred to as Sheng (victory). When C is adversely controlling A, we call this adverse control or Cheng (take advantage of). When A overcontrols C, then D is revenging by overcontrolling A and we call it Fu (revenge). These are the basic rules for disharmony in the controlling cycle. The more overcontrol there is, the more revenge there will be from D onto A.

The controlling Ke cycles and the generating Sheng cycles base themselves on the three Yin and three Yang. Tai Yang is cold and water. Yang Ming is metal and dryness. Tai Yin is earth and damp. Each element—wood, fire, earth, metal, and water—has its own use and its own life energy. The control and birth cycles of the five elements are the control and birth of these "life" energies. When we understand this principle, the application of Chinese medicine takes a different twist.

For example, when we discussed the earth element, we said that the earth is Tai Yin and its energy is damp. The Yang energy from heaven going into the earth to create the vapor of dampness is the principal way the earth comes "alive." At the same time, the earth itself is the opposite of life; the earth without Yang energy equals death. Earth plus damp will generate life, while earth with no damp will end life. This situation with the earth is of course true for the other four elements as well. When we understand this principle we realize that the generating cycle of fire giving birth to earth is actually fire generating the Yang mist of the earth, and when we talk about the wood controlling the earth, it is the wood that controls Yin (dead earth aspect). The generation cycle and the control cycle act on different aspects of the earth.

Five emotions correspond to the five elements: anger, joy, pensiveness, grief, and fear. Anger belongs to wood, joy to fire, pensiveness to earth, grief to metal, and fear to water. Within the five elements there are two types of relationships. One relationship is a nourishing (generating or giving birth) relationship, while the other is a controlling relationship.

The nourishing relationships of the emotions are anger nourishes joy, joy nourishes pensiveness, pensiveness nourishes grief, grief nourishes fear, and fear nourishes the anger again. The controlling relationships of the emotions are as follows: anger controls pensiveness, joy controls grief, pensiveness controls fear, grief controls anger, and fear controls joy.

In an emotional crisis, one must determine by observation if the emotion is in a deficient state or in an excessive state. When the emotion feels strong, the patient should sit or lie down for ten minutes to conduct the observation. If the emotion is deficient in nature, then the patient should nourish its element, and if the emotion is excessive, then the patient should control its element. For example, if grief is excessive, the patient must attempt to control the grief by increasing the amount of joy in her life, joy being the controlling emotion for grief. Because grief belongs to metal and excessive metal will overcontrol wood, controlling the grief with joy will make certain that the wood element will not suffer a great loss.

Emotions result from actions. One must think carefully his actions and then emotions are in balance. The understanding that we must follow nature in our actions is key. If we believe hearsay that following nature is unimportant and then consequently we act against nature, then our emotions are destined to be chaotic. For example, if we believe that we are our own masters and we can go to sleep whenever we want to and therefore we go to bed at 3 A.M. every morning, our emotions will have no choice but to be in disarray. If we believe that eating chemical-laden food is our personal choice, then our emotions can't be balanced. One takes actions according to nature and his emotions restore their balance naturally. Ingesting any chemicals or drugs (even antidepressants) cannot restore true balance of the emotions.

However, if the grief observed is a deficient sadness, the earth must be nourished to solve the grief, because grief is weakening the metal itself. The element that nourishes grief is pensiveness. Pensiveness is earth and earth nourishes metal. The patient should add pensiveness or thinking into her life.

It is important to keep our emotions in balance. Prolonged imbalance of the emotions will deplete the body's energy and fertility will decrease.

Inherently, emotions are neither good nor bad, they are natural. When they are out of balance, they can cause a disease, and when they're in balance, they can restore energy back to harmony. It is common to see a person who grieves for an extended period become ill, or even in extreme situations, die. It is important to

IMPAIRED EMOTION	REMEDY
Excessive anger	Sadness
Deficient anger	Fear
Excessive joy	Fear
Deficient joy	Anger
Excessive thinking	Anger
Deficient thinking	Joy
Excessive sadness	Joy
Deficient sadness	Thinking
Excessive fear	Thinking
Deficient fear	Sadness

understand the direction in which an emotion is going so we can work with it. When we know our emotions, we can remedy them.

Anger belongs to wood and its direction is upward. Anger can make us jump with clenched fists, our face becoming red as the overall energy rushes up. The power of anger is strong and intense and it has a lot of substance to it, just as does wood.

Joy is different. Its direction is also upwards, but its quality is light. When we laugh, we look up. The blood comes up to the face but the inside is hollow, or rather full of energy, with no material like fire. The fire flares upward but it is mostly energy with no physical material.

Pensiveness is even. It is in the center and it is not going up or down. Our body feels balanced and in control in this state, and we can assess our situation.

Sadness is moving down. When we grieve, we lower our heads and look downward. We sit down or lie down in the fetal position. The center of sadness is solid, like metal. We may feel like there is a lump in our throat or our chest. It feels as if something is sitting on our shoulders and pushing us down. This is the quality of metal.

Fear is also about going down. When a person is startled, he can lose control of the urine and bowels. Instead of lying down, we want to go under the bed. There is no lump in the throat or chest, but rather the knees buckle and we may feel on the verge of collapsing. The energy is fluid like water, not solid like metal. Water simply finds any way it can to flow downwards, the urine flowing without control. Everything just wants to melt down.

We need all of our emotions to stay healthy, but we must guard against emotions controlling our lives and/or impairing our health. When a relative or dear friend has died, it is good to grieve. The metal heaviness of grief is bringing you closer to the earth and helps you control the excessive anxiety coming from the liver (wood), as well as helping nourish the deficient fear coming from the kidneys (water). However, it is not good to have the emotions in excess for a long time.

How then do we know if an emotion is excessive or deficient? Excessive emotion will go with its direction, while deficient emotion will go against its direction. For anger, an excess means jumping up in anger, deficient means sitting down and clenching your teeth in anger. If the anger contains excessive wood, you flare up, and if the energy is deficient in wood, you can't flare up. With joy, excess means laughing out loud and looking upwards as you laugh, and deficient joy is laughing while looking down and covering your mouth as you laugh. For pensiveness, excess may be an inability to stop talking in order to tell other people your thoughts, and a deficiency means thinking inwardly and not sharing your constant stream of thoughts with anyone. For sadness, excess is curling in bed and crying, deficiency is to suppress the tears and feel like you can fight it, when in fact you can't. Fear excess means wanting to curl under the bed and to never come out, while fear deficiency may be a tendency to be easily startled.

When trying to balance our emotions, we need to look for the positive in each emotion. If one is angry over an IVF failure, instead of blaming the doctor or wanting to punch a hole in the wall, sit down, close your eyes and think *I am so sad I didn't get pregnant. It is no one's fault. I am just sad.* The anger will dissolve quickly and the spleen and stomach will remain undamaged. Anger is wood and wood controls earth. Stomach and spleen are earth. If the liver's anger overbears on the spleen and stomach, these two organs will become sick, very likely producing a stomach ulcer.

From my experience, at least 80 percent of infertility patients suffer kidney Yang deficiency. The emotion of the kidneys is fear. Because the emotion is excessively out of balance, the kidneys are deficient. Giving the patient hope belongs to pensiveness. The pensiveness will control excess fear and the kidneys can recover. This is why patients who are given hope sometimes become pregnant without any treatment at all.

One must have a grieving process in place when beginning a journey toward pregnancy. Fear will harm the kidneys and anger will harm the liver. When the kidneys and liver cannot function well, infertility will follow. At the same time, grief belongs to metal/lungs, and metal nourishes water/kidneys. Thus, controlled and balanced grief will help the patient strengthen the kidneys and get closer to fertility. Fear and anger are the enemies of fertility while joy, pensiveness, and grief are its friends.

···· 3 ····

CHINESE MEDICINE AND FERTILITY

Part of my inspiration to write this book comes from my experience with two particular patients, one from Chicago and the other from Hawaii, who share a common story that is not unlike many stories I have experienced in the past. The patient from Chicago was forty-four and the patient from Hawaii was forty-five. Both contacted me in early 2007. Both initially felt the Hunyuan method was too good to be true, that time was of the essence, and that more drastic measures such as IVF were needed. Both women turned away from the Hunyuan approach and went with conventional medicine. The Chicago patient tried four IVF cycles, while the Hawaiian patient tried five. Neither woman became pregnant. In early 2008, they both came back to the Hunyuan Method. Both conceived naturally, one after two months of herbal sessions, and one after five months.

Stories like these are painful for me. These women did not have to go through the IVF treatments. They did not have to spend their entire savings. They came to me first but weren't convinced I could help them. This wasn't because I didn't share success stories or the Hunyuan method didn't make sense to them, it was because they felt they couldn't go with a method that did not have the endorsement of the trillion dollar modern medicine machine.

It has been twenty-three years since I began to study Chinese medicine, and ten years since I began my research into Chinese medicine classics. This research has shed light on how to solve difficult ailments and how to grasp health. It is important to study the classics because they are the culmination of thousands of years of experience. It is not like modern "evidence-based" Western medicine, where a conclusion about a certain therapy is made within a year or two. It has been tested over many generations.

SIGNIFICANCE OF SHANG HAN (COLD INJURIES)

The *Shang Hanlun* (*Treatise about Cold Injuries*) is one of Chinese medicine's main classical works. It describes life energy, how energy works, and what we should do to make it work. Cold Injuries refer to injuries to Yang energy or an injury to the life force. In this work, author Zhang Zhongjing describes hot and cold symptoms, and shallow and deep conditions. He describes injuries to one's life force at the most initial stages and at the most terminal stages. His work encompasses the entire pathological development of one's energy.

The classical meaning of life force, or Yang energy, is warmth, while the absence of warmth is the absence of life force, thus it is called "cold injury." When the sun comes out, it is warm and when the sun is absent, it is cold. The presence of the sun gives life, while the absence of the sun eliminates life. In the same way, the presence of Yang energy gives life and the absence of Yang energy depletes life. Therefore, the absence or disturbance of Yang is referred to as a "cold injury."

In Classical Chinese Medicine, all diseases, whether hot or cold, belong to cold injuries. This is because with all illness, the life force is impaired; in other words, Yang energy is impaired. If Yang is deficient, a person will feel cold and if Yang is too localized in one spot, the person may feel hot.

Yang energy is the moving force behind life. Thus, for thousands of years, classical Chinese medicine's view was to preserve the life force Yang.

KEEPING THE YANG

Our Yang energy keeps us alive, it helps us reproduce, sleep, love, and do all the things that we accomplish in our lifetime. When we exhaust our Yang, we may feel cold, experience hot flashes, or become infertile. Stress, long hours at work, and emotional pressures can all weaken Yang energy or cause it to stagnate. Greasy, cold and depleted processed food will do so too.

However, the most significant cause of Yang deterioration is the ingestion of chemical substances. Drugs and unnatural pharmaceuticals, pesticides, preservatives in food, and pollutants in the environment should all be avoided.

The method of supporting Yang energy with herbs is a complicated art. The composition of the formulas is critical because incorrect composition will not only hinder fertility, it can also cause unnecessary side effects. I discourage patients from self-prescribing herbs or medications of any sort, for it is imperative to have had a thorough classical herbal education in order to do so.

Cold herbs are harmful to the Yang, and although they are sometimes extremely necessary, they must be used sparingly and only when needed, which is in approximately 10 percent of the time. Nevertheless, in modern herbal medicine practices, 90 percent of the patients are given cold herbs, resulting in low success rates. This is why patients and practitioners alike have little faith when it comes to infertility and herbs. In contrast, IVF seems much more successful. In my practice, however, herbal treatments are at least as successful as IVF.

Infertility patients must look for an herbalist who specializes in classical Chinese medicine. To know how to find this information, ask the practitioner about the *Shang Hanlun* theories; also, be aware of the percentage of hot herbs in the herbal formulas you are receiving. To become fertile, you need your Yang to become stronger. If you are cooling off your Yang, or exhausting it, you are drifting away from your chances of becoming pregnant.

For the infertility patient, it is important to know what is at stake if one loses Yang and how to prevent this from happening. The first step is to understand the six spheres discussed previously. The second is to shy away from cold foods, cold herbs, cold medications and cold air. The third is to control the stress, emotions, and pressures that deplete the Yang. The fourth is to refrain from hyperstimulating the Yang, either physically or emotionally.

Too much physical stimulation, such as too much exercise, will move the Yang in the Tai Yin, and too much emotion will move it in the Shao Yin. The Tai Yin organ is the spleen, which nourishes the muscles. The Tai Yin is also damp earth. Excessive Yang will dry the earth, and dry earth is dead earth. So excessive exercise will dry our earth—our bodies—and weaken our Tai Yin system. This is why many women athletes stop menstruating and become infertile.

The Shao Yin is where the kidney's water interacts with the heart's fire. The heart is where the spirit resides. When we think, contemplate, and study, we move the original Yang in the kidneys, helping the spirit revive itself. However, when we think excessively or become emotionally extended, the kidney's original Yang (water Yang) is exhausted and the spirit is lacking. This causes the water to dry, (see Yang Ming section about dry water) and the heart spirit floats.

When sexual energy is stimulated, it goes directly to the Shao Yin heart-kidney relationship. Excessive sexual mental stimulation will dry the water. Today, we can see sexually stimulating images everywhere, resulting in a numbing down of sexual desire. In contrast, in the 1950s and 1960s in China, where any reference to female sexuality was not allowed, young male villagers coming to the big city for the first time would find their pants wet from seminal emission just from riding a crowded bus. Most traditional societies and religions refrain from sex or sexual mental exploitations because free sexuality means low fertility and reduced sexual potency.

THE YANG IN THE CLASSICS

In the following section, I will quote several important Chinese medicine classics, then offer an interpretation of how they relate to infertility.

THE TREATISE OF ANCIENT TIMES AND THE HEAVENLY TRUTH:

> The ancient sages knew the right path to longevity. They followed the rules of Yin and Yang and they harmonized themselves with the help of numbers. They well regulated their diet and sleeping habits and they never exhausted themselves. Because of this, their bodies and spirits thrived and they fulfilled their life expectancy. They lived to be more than one hundred and then they passed away. Today's people are not the same. Harmful drinks are their nectar and exhausting themselves is the routine. They indulge in their desires, exhausting their essence and scattering their true Yang. Today's people don't know how to keep their energy full; they don't know how to regulate their spirit. They want to make their heart happy instead of true happiness. Even the sleep is not regulated and that is why they reach the age of fifty and their body has greatly declined.

This quote is from the very first chapter of *The Yellow Emperor*. The main message is that we should all strive for healthier lives because it will enable us to fulfill our destiny, and allow women to become pregnant at the oldest possible age. Furthermore, this chapter introduces the concept of living in harmony according to the Yin and Yang. It tells us how to regulate our diet, as well as how to guard against exhausting our essence and scattering our true Yang.

THE GREAT TREATISE OF THE FOUR SEASONS AND REGULATING THE QI AND SPIRIT:

The three months of spring is when the old is expelled and new is born. The heaven and earth are born and the myriad things flourish. You should go to sleep late and wake up early. This is the right time to start exercising. It is also the right time to start thinking and planning as the energy spreads out and does not stagnate. In this season, there is only birth and no death, and there is only prosperity with no decline. This is the right path to nurture on the birthing energy of the spring. If you go against it, you will harm your liver. Your summer's energy will turn cold and the glory of summer will be scanty.

The three months of summer are referred to as "full glory." The heaven and earth are in full exchange and the myriad things are in full glory. You should go to sleep late and wake up early. Do not feel bitter that the days are long and make sure that your mind is free of anger. Allow your spirit to flourish and your energy to expand as if the things that you love are all outside of your body. This is the right path to nurture on the summer's expanding energy. If you go against it, you will harm your heart.

The three months of fall are referred to as "to even out." The heaven's winds are blowing and the earth colors are changing. You should go to sleep early and wake up early following the rooster. Calm your mind and be peaceful as to join the fall's quieting down energy. Gather inward your energy and spirit as to match the fall's descending energy. Not thinking outward will cause the lung's energy to be clear. If you go against this path, you will harm your lungs. Your winter's energy will suffer drainage and the storage of winter will be scanty.

The three months of winter are called the storage. The water is ice and the earth is dry. One must follow the sunlight and go to sleep early and wake up late. All thoughts and desires should be directed inwards. Nothing should be radiating outward. Although it is important to dispel the external cold and keep warm, perspiration must be avoided. The Yang energy must be allowed to sink in deep. Going against this path will result in harm to the kidneys. The spring energy will suffer cold and infertility and the birth energy of spring will be scanty.

The main principle for maintaining health, according to the Yellow Emperor, is conforming to nature. Our behavior and actions should change every season according to the state of Yang energy around us.

When Yang energy expands in summer, we should allow our energy to expand, and when the energy moves into storage in winter, we should follow as well. This includes many aspects of our lives: the way we sleep, eat, exercise, think, and express ourselves. For example, in the summer we should be outgoing and social, while in winter more inward looking and reserved. In the summer, we should sleep shorter hours, in winter we should sleep longer.

Our primary strategy to gain fertility is not with herbs or acupuncture, and certainly not drugs and surgeries. We should adjust our sleep, food, stress, emotions, and everything else according to the changes of Yang in the four seasons.

THE TREATISE ON LIFE'S ENERGY CONFORMING TO HEAVEN:

> The most crucial aspect of Yin and Yang is that the Yang must become dense and consolidate. If Yin and Yang don't harmonize, it is like the spring without the fall, or the winter without the summer. When the two harmonize, it is called "the way of the sage." If the Yang "opening" is too strong and it can't condense into storage, then the Yin energy will perish. When Yin is peaceful and Yang can withdraw back into storage, then the spirit is thriving. When Yin and Yang separate, our energy will extinguish.

This section explains the importance of Yang within our energy. Yang gives us the ability to function, and even more importantly, it has the ability and need to withdraw back into storage. If Yang can't withdraw, then Yin energy will perish. Yin energy is the energy within the matter—within every cell—of our body. When the Yin energy has perished, our life will become shorter. Over-stimulation will cause Yang to expand and not withdraw back. This can be overstimulation of the mind, or physical stimulation from coffee, smoking, or drugs. This is the reason many infertility patients suffer night sweats after taking fertility drugs. Yang is expanded and is unable to retreat into storage, prompting Yin to begin to perish.

THE GREAT TREATISE OF YIN AND YANG REFLECTIONS:

> With strong heat, the energy will decline, while with
> mild warmth the energy will grow stronger. Strong
> heat is feeding on the energy, while the energy is
> feeding on mild warmth. Strong heat will scatter the
> energy, while mild warmth will give birth to energy.

This segment explains the principle of balance, a key point in
Chinese medicine. Warmth is beneficial, while strong heat can
be destructive. This concept of keeping in balance is true for all
aspects of life—diet, exercise, sleep—even for reproductive endo-
crinology.

In order to know where the correct balance lies, we must look
to nature and the wisdom of our forefathers. Most scientific "new"
ideas are here today and gone tomorrow. What is advised with
confidence one year is reversed the next. I will continue to believe
in the ancient wisdom of longevity and health when it comes to
diet, exercise, sleep, and treatment.

> A healer with great skill will treat a problem when
> it first arises at the superficial level of the skin. If he
> is too late, he will treat the disease at the flesh level.
> If he has missed it even more, he will treat it at the
> tendons and meridians depth. If the disease has
> formed already and the healer is late, he will treat it
> at the six Yang organs. If he has no choice and the
> disease has established itself in the depths, he can only
> treat it at the five Yin organs. When the disease gets to
> the deep level of the five Yin organs, it is a situation
> called "half alive and half dead." There can be only
> partial recovery.

The wisdom of Chinese medicine is far reaching. The Yellow Emperor explains that the true remedy of all disease is prevention. But if not prevented, it is best to treat a disease early and correctly while it is at the skin, or superficial, level.

Every disease has a path of deterioration and a path of recovery. Regarding diet, sleep, stress, and treatment of any kind, the correct measure will lead to recovery and the wrong measure creates disharmony and deterioration. Treating a disease which has penetrated into the five Yin organs, however, is a difficult task and can ensure only partial recovery.

When a patient receives Western drugs, symptoms are removed from the exterior level, but are pushed inward into the five Yin organs. It is often difficult for the patient to discontinue the medication because of drug dependencies; the inner organs cannot function properly by themselves anymore.

THE GRAND TREATISE OF ESSENTIALS OF THE ULTIMATE TRUTH:

The Yellow Emperor asked: "I know that the five weather phenomena interact with each other and there are excesses and deficiencies and that the six spheres take their place to rule the heaven and earth. What is the significance of all this?" Qibo bowed and answered: "This is the big principle of heaven and earth and it reflects into the human spirit." The Emperor said: "I heard that in heaven this principle unites with the mysterious and on earth it joins with the unexplained. Why is that so?" Qibo answered: "This is how the right path is born. This is also where ignorant doctors become suspicious."

The five weather transformations of nature and the six spheres are a reflection of the human body. When we conform to this big principle, we can say that we follow the right path. The problem is that much of this principle is concealed in the mysterious ways of nature, and we as humans are uncomfortable with this mystery. We want to know why things happen. Our instinct is to understand nature so we can conquer it and not be conquered by it. Physicians who don't quite understand the "right path" nature is creating become suspicious of it, and ultimately come up with their own path, which does not conform to nature.

THE TREATISE OF TRANSFORMING ESSENCE AND ENERGY:

> The Emperor asked: "I heard that in ancient times the sages could heal and transform essence and energy by using a blessing. In today's world, we use herbs to heal the inside of the body and acupuncture to heal the outside. Sometimes, the patient recovers and sometimes not. Why is this so?" Qibo answered: "The sages lived among the animals. Their actions were tuned to avoid cold and their shelter protected them from extreme heat. Their emotions never harmed them internally and the external world never exhausted their physical body. Because of their harmonious lifestyle, a disease could not penetrate deep. In today's world, the story is different. Emotions harm our insides and the external world inflicts great damage upon our body. We do not follow the four seasons and we don't care to protect ourselves from cold and extreme heat. Diseases of all sorts attack us and penetrate deep from the skin to the bone marrow. Every little disease becomes a big one and every big disease results in death. This is why a little blessing cannot heal anymore and we need the use of herbs and acupuncture."

"The ancient sages lived among the animals" means that the sages lived in harmony with nature as the animals do. They were in tune with the four seasons and understood the state of Yang energy in each season, and how it affects daily life. When we live in accord with nature, emotions come and go very easily; they cannot harm us. We do not hold grudges nor hold onto fear for extended periods of time. It is similar to a storm: the emotions of the sky are discharged gracefully and the sun comes out immediately thereafter.

It is difficult to let go of the fear of infertility. When Western physicians instill this fear into their patients, it tends to stay with the woman and harms her chances even further by harming the kidneys' ability to hold the essence. If you live according to nature, this fear comes and goes quickly.

In addition, the sages made sure that the external world would not harm their physical bodies. The external world is composed of two parts: our lifestyle and the external factors around us. We shouldn't subject ourselves to extreme temperatures, nor should we eat cold foods. Many of my patients report sitting entire days in a freezing office during their workweek. Other patients take supplements because it is difficult to find the healthiest of foods.

First educate yourself about nature and how it impacts your life, making it short or long, wasting your Yang or not, then set up your priorities: Is my Yang more important or is the job, is my life more important or what modern prejudice of health is more important? If your life is the most important to you, then rearrange priorities. Your modern world is the world you create. Eating healthy, sleeping early, not allowing your job to dominate your life, and so forth, are all personal choices, they seem to be dictated by society but in reality every person dictates them to himself. At the end of the day one should never blame society or bad situations, only the choices that one made during his lifetime.

We should, however, set priorities. The first and foremost is to keep our health, even if it means another job in a warmer office, or spending more time locating the correct food. We should not suffer through anything when it comes to our health, because everything else is secondary. We must attempt to sleep longer hours, eat warmer foods, and exercise less in the winter to ensure that our kidney's energy will stay in surplus.

Additional influences are diseases that attack us and penetrate deep into the "bone marrow." This is not a literal description, but rather an expression describing depth on the energy level scale. If our body is strong, illnesses cannot go into a deep energetic level, but if our body is weak, then an illness can go deep. Another reason a disease can go deep is using the wrong treatment. When we become ill and take a drug to alleviate the symptom, this will push the disease deeper into a "bone marrow" depth. This is because a symptom is not a disease. When the true root of a disease, rather than a symptom, is remedied, then the disease will be cured.

For example, if one doesn't sleep enough in winter, the lower back may become sore because the kidneys' energy is exhausted. If pain medication is taken to resolve the lower backache, the pain might be temporarily relieved, but the kidneys are still exhausted and the sleep patterns are still off. The pain alarm that signals that the kidneys are deficient of energy is no longer felt. Later on, a severe disease surfaces and nobody knows why. This is why the Yellow Emperor says: "Every small disease becomes a big one." In Chinese medicine treatment, the practitioner must strengthen the kidneys and advise the patient to sleep more during this season. This is a true remedy. The root is treated and the cause for the root problem is being addressed.

Western medicine has tried to adapt a preventative approach. The tracking of cholesterol and triglyceride levels has given birth to new drugs aimed at "preventing" heart disease. However, these discoveries are all man-made and not derived from nature. My experience shows that following nature's rhythm results in unsurpassable health, and more importantly, it comes for free as an entitlement. We are part of nature and nature is part of us. Drugs for preventative reasons are unnecessary if one knows how to follow the path.

THE TREATISE ON PRECIOUS LIFE AND THE ENTIRE FORM:

> First you must control the spirit, second you must know how to nourish the body, third you must know the real truth about "toxic" herbs, fourth you must know the ins and outs of acupuncture, and fifth you must know how to understand and diagnose the inner organ patterns, the blood and energy. When you know all of the above, the right path is not mysterious anymore. It is open in front of you, but you may be alone on this path.

The first element needed to pursue the correct path toward health, longevity, and fertility is to control the spirit, meaning to conform to nature and the six spheres. The second principle is to nourish the body. The third, fourth, and fifth principles of keeping healthy and following the right path are to know the truth about herbs, acupuncture, and the art of diagnosis. The three combined represent the art of Chinese medicine. It explains that once your vibration matches the vibration of nature and you understand how nature works, you can use all natural resources such as herbs, grains, fruits, meats, and vegetables to nurture your body. If you have failed the natural path to health and become ill, you should know how to assess and treat your illness using herbs and acupuncture remedies.

THE TREATISE ON STORING THE ENERGY AND LIVING ACCORDING TO THE SEASONS:

> Toxic herbs can defeat a disease, the five grains will nurture, the five fruits will help, the five meats will benefit and the five vegetables will supplement. The energy and flavor of each will unite and enter the body. This will strengthen your essence and benefit your energy.

Ingesting only natural foods and herbs is called nourishing the body. We must differentiate, however, between what is produced by nature and many other products that are labeled "natural."

TREATISE ABOUT PAINS:

> The Yellow Emperor said: "I heard that the one who knows the heaven rules must have good knowledge of people. The one who knows the ancient times

95

must have good knowledge of the present, and the one who knows people must know himself well. In this way, the right path cannot be lost and the truth comes out. This is called true understanding."

To truly understand the right path for health, one must understand the heaven's energies, the wisdom accumulated in the past, and most of all, one must cultivate character and know oneself. It is important that we choose a way of self-cultivation, such as meditation, Tai Chi, Qi Gong or Yoga.

DISCUSSION OF PULSE ESSENTIALS:

The Emperor asked: "What is the method of diagnosis?" Qibo answered: "Diagnosis is done early in the morning, before the Yin Qi moved and before the Yang Qi scattered, before any food or drink entered the mouth and the energy in the meridians surged. The meridians at this time are still in order and the Qi and blood are not yet chaotic. At this time you can diagnose the excess of the pulse."

What does "scatter" mean? The Chinese character for "scatter" is composed of three parts. The first is hemp fiber or a stack of wood, the second flesh, and third a component showing a beating action. All the components brought together mean that beating on a stack of wood, hemp fiber or flesh will cause it to break apart. The Yang action is then to break apart. What is Yang breaking from? It is breaking from the flesh to go outward. What is Yin doing? It is giving the momentum to the Yang to go out. When the Yang is silent or in storage, it cannot go out or break out. The Yin has the force to push this weight out. When the Yang is closing down, the Yin is also resting. They are actually not different from each other, but two sides of the same coin. The Yin is moving the momentum and the Yang is breaking out. That is why the Yellow Emperor says: "The knowledgeable sees the sameness and the fool sees the difference. The knowledgeable always has plenty and the fool is always in deficiency."

STIMULATING DRUGS AND THE YANG DON'T ALWAYS MIX

Although Western fertility drugs are considered safe, I believe it is important to remember that certain drugs, which were initially found to be safe, were later found to be harmful. Such a drug was DES (Diethylstilboestrol), a synthetic estrogen that was prescribed by both obstetricians and general practitioners to millions of pregnant women in many countries from 1938 through the 1980s. Thought to prevent miscarriage and ensure a healthy pregnancy, over two hundred brand names of this drug were sold; it never worked well and was eventually found to pose health risks, such as cancer and infertility, to the women who took the drug and the children they carried.

Patients who have had IVF treatments often come to me with a serious Yang deficiency caused by the overstimulating drugs, and/or the cold herbs they've been taking. Stimulating drugs of any sort, including fertility drugs, stimulate the Yang to come out of the water. Their symptoms range from cold hands and feet, to feeling cold all over, to general exhaustion and repeated hot flashes. In addition to herbal supplements, I recommend seeking help from a qualified practitioner instead of purchasing herbal supplements from a health food store.

Infertility is becoming more prevalent as Yang deficiencies increase in the population. Zheng Qinan in his book *True Transmission of Chinese Medicine Theory* (*Yi Li Zhen Chuan*) explains that: "The true Yang resides below and penetrates the Yin. If the true fire is weak, it cannot control the lower orifices, blood and essence. When the true fire is weak, the Yin rises upwards, which can cause shortness of breath and a floating pulse. However, if the face is not red, the body is not hot and there is no sweat, then the true Yang is not rising with the Yin (which is a good prognosis). However, if there is red face, the body feels hot and there is sweating, then the true Yang is floating and truly wants to separate from the Yin (this is a bad prognosis)."

I have witnessed the deterioration of true Yang in the kidneys of patients taking fertility drugs. Symptoms include hot flashes and night sweats. These hurt the body by hurting Yang energy, which is responsible for conception and pregnancy; it also lessens fertility potential.

Even though my position on fertility drugs is generally negative, I am not opposed to their use. I have spent hundreds of hours in a Western fertility clinic as part of my doctoral program, and witnessed the miracles that fertility drugs can achieve. I have seen patients with deformed uteruses, abnormal ovaries and other anatomical situations, who would never have been able to give birth if it weren't for modern tecŸology and drugs. I know that Western doctors, especially many reproductive endocrinologists, are passionate, kindhearted, and want to help their patients get pregnant.

The problem is not with the doctors or even with the drugs. The problem is with Western medicine as a whole because it does not allow any other treatment modality to penetrate into the health care system. Due to public pressure, the system is finally changing now. Acupuncture has begun to be accepted in some medical circles. Its efficacy is well documented, yet, as recently as five years ago, most reproductive endocrinologists would not have referred their patients to an acupuncturist.

There is still a long way to go. Most patients who want to get pregnant don't have Chinese medicine as an option. Most Western doctors do not refer their patients to herbalists, and patients who try Chinese medicine usually discover it themselves.

This must change. It makes sense to inflict less damage on the patient. IVF procedures are useless in patients with Yang deficiencies. Because they only work in patients with a strong Yang, the deficiency must be remedied before IVF procedures are attempted. Except in extreme cases, infertility patients should be treated first via Chinese medicine, and if that doesn't work, move onto fertility drugs and IVF.

One reproductive endocrinologist who is a collaborator of mine tries to improve the health of his patients for the first six months, and if the patient has not conceived at that point, he begins the "shotgun approach" of fertility drugs. Unfortunately, such doctors are definitely the exception rather than the rule. I believe that twenty or thirty years from now, Chinese herbal medicine will be assimilated into the Western medicine dogma the very same way acupuncture is today. However, for today's generation of patients, there is no time to wait.

THE GREAT TREATISE OF YIN AND YANG REFLECTIONS:

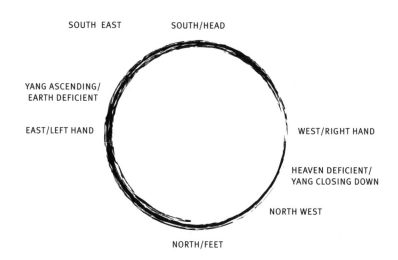

"Heaven is deficient in north and west and the man's right ear and right eye are not as clear as the left ear and eye. Earth is not full at south east so the man's left hand and left foot are not as strong as the right hand and right foot. The east is Yang. The Yang's essence is to ascend upwards. If it is at the upper part of the body, then it is bright and not deficient on that side. This is where the heaven and earth, Yin and Yang cannot be complete."

If we look at the same energy circle we have previously explored, we can understand the Yellow Emperor's statements. Our head is at the south or heaven, and our feet are in the north or earth; the right side of our body is in the west and the left side of our body is in the east. Because the Yang energy is stronger on the left, as its essence is going upward, the left eye and left ear are stronger than the right. The right eye and ear are on the side where Yang energy descends, so they are lacking energy in comparison to the left. The eyes, ears, and nose deal with Yang clear energy. There is no physical substance coming in and out of them, only energy, be it sunlight, sound waves, or air.

The hands and feet are different. They deal with substance and materials. They need Yin energy—the energy of the earth—to help them. The Yin and earth are deficient at the southeast, where Yang is most active. Yin and earth are the strongest where the Yang is closing down (Northwest), thus the right hand and foot are stronger.

The five Yin organs: heart, spleen, lungs, kidneys, and liver, store the essences of the five directions. The five essences are the essences of heaven and earth. The five directions characterize the essences: east, south, west, north, and center.

Discussion on Golden Chamber's True Words:

> East has green color and it enters the liver, it opens to
> the eyes and stores its essence in the liver. Its ailment
> is trembling (Jing He), its flavor sour, its kind grass

and trees, its animal chicken and its grain wheat. This is the spring, which is coming first. Its sound is Jue, its number is eight. The illness, you should know, is at the tendons. Its smell is rank.

South has the color red, it enters the heart and opens into the ears, its essence is stored in the heart. Because of this, its disease is in the five Yin organs. Its flavor is bitter and its kind fire. Its animal is sheep and its grain broomcorn millet. You should know that its diseases are in the blood vessels. Its sound is Zheng and its number seven. Its smell is burnt.

Center has the color yellow, it enters the spleen, opens to the mouth and its essence is stored in the spleen. Because of this, diseases are in the root of the tongue. Its animal is ox and its grain millet. You should know that its disease is in the flesh. Its sound is Gong and its number five. Its smell is fragrant.

West has the color white, it enters the lungs and opens into the nose. Its essence is stored in the lungs. Its disease is in the shoulders, its flavor pungent and its kind metal, its animal horse and its grain rice. You should know that its disease is in the skin and body hair. Its sound is Shang and its number nine. Its smell is rancid.

North has black color. It enters the kidneys and opens into the two Yin (anus and genitalia). Its essence is stored in the kidneys. Its disease is at Xi (the connection between the small muscles and bones). Its flavor is salty and its kind water, its animal pig and its grain beans. You should know that its disease is in the bones. Its sound is Yu and its number six. Its smell is rotten.

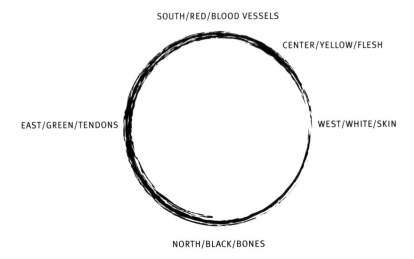

SOUTH/RED/BLOOD VESSELS

CENTER/YELLOW/FLESH

EAST/GREEN/TENDONS

WEST/WHITE/SKIN

NORTH/BLACK/BONES

The five directions have distinct colors. The colors are the manifestation of the heaven's energies. The red color feels hot, the green feels warm like spring, yellow is like the end of summer transforming hot to cool, white is cool and similar to the fall, and black is cold like the winter. These colors or energies are natural expressions of Yin and Yang.

The colors/energies are present in our body from our conception, when our father and mother mix their colors together and give it to us.

The quality of the colors, as the Yellow Emperor says, has

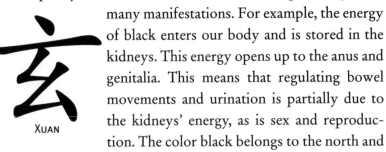

XUAN

many manifestations. For example, the energy of black enters our body and is stored in the kidneys. This energy opens up to the anus and genitalia. This means that regulating bowel movements and urination is partially due to the kidneys' energy, as is sex and reproduction. The color black belongs to the north and it belongs to water. North, water, and black possess the same energy. Black in the Chinese language is Xuan, which not only translates to "black," but to "mysterious" as well.

Looking at the classical meaning of Xuan in the earliest Chinese dictionary tells us that the color is conceived of black with a hint of red. Red is fire or Yang energy and black is water or Yin energy. The black energy of the kidneys embodies the seed of Yang—the seed of a new life. This is what we referred to as the energy of Shao Yin in the three Yin/three Yang system.

The Yellow Emperor goes further to explain that colors shape everything physical around us. The animals, the grains, the flavors and even our own body tissues, are all an expression of these colors. The quality of the black color, for example, is the core reason why our bones have formed the way they did, and the white color or white energy explains our skin. When we understand that, we can understand the holistic view of Chinese medicine. If, let's say, a patient has a disease of the tendons, we will treat the liver. The liver stores the essence of the green energy in the body, which is the same energy responsible for the formation of tendons. When the liver energy grows strong, the tendons can heal.

The same is true with most infertility issues. The reproductive system is weak because the black (with hint of red) is not sufficient. We strengthen the kidneys so the black energy of the body will become strong. When the black energy is strong, the sperm is good and the egg quality is at its best. If a physician refers to "poor egg quality" it signals that the black energy is not strong enough.

The energy of the five colors and five directions is the energy of heaven and earth. The heaven's energy comes down to interact with the earth and provides the earth with energy. This is called Qi Jiao, the space between heaven and earth where humans, animals, plants, and

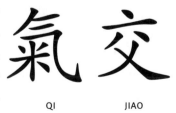

QI   JIAO

trees live. The five colors or energies must follow a correct path for harmony to exist. The same is true with the five energies inside our body. They must follow a correct path or disease will result.

So, for example, black energy is the strongest after midnight in the very early hours of the new day. If a couple has intercourse at this time, but the black energy is deficient, pregnancy will be impossible. It does not help if the black energy is strong in the middle of the day, when it shouldn't be. If the black energy is strong in the middle of the day, one feels tired, which will hinder conception.

Chinese medicine is not fixed like Western medicine. A Western diagnosis of "poor egg quality" means poor egg quality whether it is day or night, winter or spring. Chinese medicine recognizes that energy fluctuates in different times in different ways, represented by the different colors. My experience and results show that poor egg quality is not necessarily poor at all. When colors are deficient or when they are not in harmony, namely at the wrong place at the wrong time, the woman cannot get pregnant, and the quality of the egg does not matter. When the energies restore harmony, the woman will get pregnant even with "poor egg quality."

The Yellow Emperor explains that in the Qi Jiao, during the energy interaction between heaven and earth, six actions are occurring simultaneously: virtue, transformation, affair, effect, extreme change, and a possible disaster. These actions are happening between heaven and earth, but they also reflect in our body.

The Yellow Emperor tells us that to understand harmony and become fertile, we must understand how energies work. The energies of nature and of our body, reflected from nature, have normal functions and expressions. These energies also undergo extreme changes and disasters, making it impossible for the body to function correctly. Infertility is one issue arising due to such a change of energy. As many as 89 percent of my patients complain of feeling cold and having cold hands and feet, which is due to extreme change or even a disaster in the kidneys. The kidneys, water, and the black color are in trouble. If I succeed in alleviating this problem of extreme change, the patient conceives. The black color will become harmonious and the patient will become pregnant. However, if the black color does not harmonize, neither the patient's youth nor her state of "perfect health" will enable her to become pregnant naturally through medical tecÿology.

This principle seems simple; however, in reality it is not. Even though most patients feel cold, it is not always the fault of the black color. There are other colors as well. The heaven's energies and the patient's body energies must be in balance. The art of Chinese medicine is first to recognize what is out of balance, then how to restore it. Because the essences of heaven and earth energies are stored inside our organs, the practitioner must know what is going on in nature daily. If he does not, he will not understand "reflections," and the treatment results will be poor.

The Yellow Emperor says, "The emperor asked: 'There must be rules for the use of acupuncture.' Qibo answered: 'One must follow the heaven's rules and the principles of earth, unite the two until they shine bright. As for the method of acupuncture, one must first map out the stars and the moon, and know the seasons and the eight current energies. Only then can one utilize acupuncture. If the heaven is warm, the blood is flowing and the Qi is floating. If the heaven is cold, the blood is coagulating and the Qi sinks. When the moon has just begun to grow, the blood and Qi are thin and narrow in essence, and when the moon is full, the blood and Qi are full and the flesh is firm. When the moon is on the decline, the flesh decreases its firmness and the meridians are empty."

In the past few years, there have been studies showing both the benefits of acupuncture for IVF, as well as those showing that acupuncture actually decreased IVF success. There is no answer, because to study acupuncture scientifically is wrong.

In the context of "reflections," the Yellow Emperor explains that the characteristics of the individual under treatment, as well as the season, moon phase, and time of day, will all affect the location of acupuncture points, the length of the needles, and how these needles will be twisted.

The Yellow Emperor –Miraculous Pivot states: "If you want to use acupuncture, you must first inspect the meridians to see if they are full or empty. You palpate the channel and follow its path; you press and knead it to find out its condition. Then you must look for the reflections. Only then can you choose which meridian to use and where to put the needles."

This explains that each acupuncture patient must be checked carefully. Each meridian has to be observed and analyzed. Thereafter, the practitioner must study the current reflections of heaven in the body. These reflections change constantly. When heaven changes, the reflections also change. Only then can the practitioner choose the meridians, needles, acupuncture points, and correct tecŸique.

THE GREAT TREATISE OF YIN AND YANG REFLECTIONS:
"Strong fire causes the Qi to decline, while mild warmth strengthens the Qi. Strong fire consumes the Qi, while Qi feeds on mild warmth. Strong fire scatters Qi, while mild warmth gives birth to Qi."

When we study Western medicine pathology, we learn that bacteria or viruses trigger numerous diseases. This includes meningitis, prostatitis, herpes and other illnesses. However, bacteria and viruses are often present in the body even though no illness has occurred. The viruses and bacteria attack or colonize only in selected people.

The above quote from *The Yellow Emperor* explains how the pathogens choose their victims. The principle that mild warmth nourishes the Qi is as true for culturing embryos for IVF as it is for culturing bacteria to make yogurt. If the temperature is very cold or very hot, nothing will happen. The temperature must be appropriately warm for the culture to grow.

The same is true inside the body with regard to reproduction. Warmth is the green energy of spring and the energy of the liver in the Jue Yin (see chapter two). This green energy cannot translate into external temperature. This is an internal temperature that must be reached in the right place at the right time. Any woman who has charted her body's basal temperature knows that temperatures fluctuate during the menstrual cycle and ovulation. However, the temperature is only one aspect of green warmth. The other aspect of warmth (green) is its gentle spreading out, which occurs if the green essence of heaven is stored appropriately in the liver. This helps us understand why so many infertile women feel cold, and why bacteria and viruses attack some people and not others. It is the result of imbalances of reflected energy. It is not warm enough nor is it too hot, it is not cool enough nor is it too cold. This causes pathogens to move to one place or another, to attack one person and not another. This happens because the reflection and absorption of reflections is not harmonious.

The Yellow Emperor advises practitioners to treat the cause and not the symptoms. The root of the problem is disharmony in reflections, resulting from disharmony in the heavens or from an internal disharmony, such as emotions, that obstruct the body from absorbing reflections correctly. The practitioner's job is to know the heavens and the internal causes. He should look for the cause and cure it. Often patients tell me "you are a miracle worker." In reality, assisting my patients to become healthy has very little to do with miracles. It rather has to do with knowledge. Even though this knowledge is not easy to come by (it's not always in textbooks), it is worthwhile to invest the extra effort to attain it.

THE FEMALE ENERGY – BY THE LIGHT OF THE MOON

TREATISE OF THE EIGHT MAIN SECTIONS AND A CLEAR SPIRIT:
"When the moon begins to grow, the blood and energy begin forming essence and the protective energy starts moving. When the moon is full, the blood and energy are full and the body's flesh is solid. When the moon is empty, the flesh decreases its firmness, the meridians are relatively empty, the protective energy is missing and the physical body is stripped of energy.

"One must recognize these heavenly changes and then regulate the blood and energy accordingly. When the heaven is cold, avoid cold acupuncture, and when the heaven is warm, avoid moxa-bustion (burning of herbs). When the moon is growing, avoid reducing methods and when the moon is full, avoid tonifying methods. When the moon is empty, do not treat (tonify or reduce, use only even methods) and this is called following the changes of heaven in harmonizing the patient."

Why is the female menstrual cycle one moon long? This is a question related to Yin and Yang. If we take our world and mix into it an energetic polarity, we get life. Life is a constant mixture of two polarities, like the plus and minus of electricity. There is a man and a woman and when the two are brought together, life results. But what makes a man Yang and what makes a woman Yin? Is it because the man received a Y chromosome and the woman didn't? Is that just a coincidence?

Chinese medicine does not believe in "coincidences." There is a reason for everything, even if we don't understand why. *The Yellow Emperor* calls it "the mysterious way of heaven." But when one analyzes this mystery, one can see many things, including an obvious polarity. The day turns into night and the night turns into day. The summer turns into winter and the winter turns into summer. The male has genitalia, which are meant to give, and the female has genitalia that are meant to receive.

Lao Zi wrote in the chapter "Four Infinities" of the Chinese classic *Dao De Jing*:

> Before the World exists
> Much is mysterious:
> Quiet, depthless,
> Solitary, unchanging,
> Everywhere and ever moving,
> The mother of the World.
> I do not know its name, so I call it Dao;
> I do not know its limit, so I call it infinite.

Lao Zi uses the description "mother of the world" to describe the energy responsible for creating this world—a feminine energy first captured by the moon. Just like a woman receiving the male's essence, or sperm, the moon is the recipient of the sunlight Yang energy. The growth of this Yang fullness, coming concurrently with the changes of the moon, is the time when the "mysterious" happens and a new life is created. The times of the moon are, as previously discussed, the times of the three Yin: Tai Yin, Shao Yin, and Jue Yin. A new Yin energy is born as the Yang energy goes into rest. These are the times where we end the life of one day, going to sleep for the night. The moon—the mother of the world—then births us into the dawn of a new life.

> The female receives her energy from the moon—the reflection of the sun's Yang energy, which we call Yin energy. So in *Treatise of the Eight Main Sections and a Clear Spirit*, Qibo writes: "When the moon starts growing, the blood and energy start forming essence and the protective energy starts moving. When the moon is full, the blood and energy are full and the body's flesh is solid. When the moon is empty, the flesh decreases its firmness, the meridians are rela-

tively empty, the protective energy is missing and the physical body is stripped of energy. One must recognize the above heavenly changes and regulate the blood and energy accordingly."

The woman's blood and energy conform to the moon and increase in volume when the moon is full, allowing the Yang essence to enter. Her energy decreases when the moon is empty and Yin takes over. This is the same principle that causes the water in the sea to rise and sink with low and high tides. The increase in blood and energy when the moon is full allows the Yang essence to enter.

If during the menstrual cycle the Yang essence is introduced into the female and a new Yang is born, the Yin energy will continue to flourish and attach to the new baby, which is a pregnancy. However, if the Yang is not introduced, or if it is introduced but no new Yang is born, the Yin will increase and energy will decline. All the extra Yin energy amassed during the first and second halves of the cycle is discharged out of the body. This is the menses: the extra Yin energy for which the woman's body no longer has any use. Yang has declined and Yin energy goes with it into hiding. During a pregnancy where the Yang continues to grow, the woman's Yin and blood can double or even triple, ensuring the baby's ability to attract Yang.

The woman's menstrual cycle follows the moon movements in the increase and decrease of Yin energy. It increases to receive Yang and decreases when there is no new Yang created. It is the best example to show that our body vibrates in accord with nature.

Why don't all women menstruate when the moon is empty? Our bodies are impacted by a variety of factors in addition to the moon, and it is even more so because we have distanced ourselves from nature. Because of external and internal influences, some women start their cycle before the moon starts its birth and others start their cycle thereafter. A few of my patients tell me that they menstruate like clockwork every time the moon is full or empty, but most women do not conform to this pattern to an exact degree. However, it is clear that the menstrual cycle, at twenty-eight days, is one moon long. When the body is in disharmony with the moon, the period can come every fourteen days or every two months, or even not at all. According to the Yellow Emperor, the menstrual cycle stops after seven cycles of seven years, or after forty-nine years. At this point, natural fertility stops and the woman's Yin does not increase and decline with the lunar cycles.

It is important to understand here that the menstrual cycle is not the result of the uterus "wanting" to shed its lining. It is rather because the body is conforming to nature and to the lunar movements. This closeness with nature is important to understand, because if conventional medicine theory is followed instead, birth control pills and/or fertility drugs will induce menstruation at odd times. This will distort the Yin cycles of the body, taking the patient further away from giving birth to a new Yang. This is not what Lao Zi calls "the mother of the world."

Of course, Western medicine does not recognize the relationship between the female menses and the lunar cycles. Why? As *The Great Treatise of Essentials of the Ultimate Truth* states: "*The Yellow Emperor* asked: 'I know that the five weather phenomena interact with each other and there are excesses and deficiencies (lunar surge and decline) and that the six spheres take their place to rule the heaven and earth. What is the significance of all this?' Qibo bowed and answered: 'This is the big principle of heaven and earth and it reflects into the human spirit.' The emperor said: 'I heard that in heaven this principle unites with the mysterious and on earth it joins with the unexplained. Why is that so?' Qibo answered: 'This is how the right path is born. This is also the reason why uneducated doctors become suspicious.'"

MALE AND FEMALE UNITE

The man's energy comes from the sun, while the woman's energy comes from the moon. The menstrual cycle is a Yin action, and its implication is to receive the Yang. The Yin action occurs in the lower part of the body, also called the lower heater. This includes the uterus, kidneys, and liver. The man's desire to reproduce is the Yang action. It happens in the upper part of the body, also called the upper heater. This includes the heart, head, and lungs.

THE GREAT TREATISE OF YIN AND YANG REFLECTIONS:
"Yin and Yang are the paths of heaven and earth, it is the reason for everything on earth, it is the mother and father of transformation, it is the root of birth and decline, it is the palace of the clear spirit."

The relationship and harmony of Yin and Yang happens on many different levels. Some levels are physical while some are spiritual. Some levels are easy to understand while some are difficult.

NOTE TO THE READER:
This discussion of spiritual and physical levels may be difficult to understand. It may require more than one reading. If you come across a section that is vague and/or obscure, please leave it behind and read further. Later on, you can go back to it.

NINE MONTHS PREGNANCY – THE SECRET OF LIFE AND DEATH

Pregnancy is the story of life and death, two events which are very much dependent on each other. In Chinese medicine, this dependency is referred to as the secret of life and death.

In today's mechanical world, we believe that a sperm enters an egg, then chromosomes unite and the cells begin to divide. A fetus develops out of this mutation—arms and legs, brain, heart, and other organs—and we have a baby.

I believe that pregnancy, which is life and death, carries a different story. It is a story of a dying man, one who lived to the age of eighty, lived his life to its fullest, and sired many children who produced many grandchildren. This man had many stories throughout his life. How he loved and hated, worked for many years to support his family, and how his eyes filled with tears of joy as he saw his children become successful and have their own children. On his deathbed, this handsome man of life battled a grave disease of death. As life was running out, his wishes and desires began to change. He saw no use for clothes, food, and entertainment. His only desires were to enjoy the warm morning sun and sip water.

As we already know, the circle explains much of Chinese medicine's understanding of life and death, of pregnancy and birth. The east is where the sun rises and the west is where the sun descends. The east is where spring begins and the west is where fall enters into storage. The east is where the morning begins and the west is where the evening descends.

As previously explained, the east and west ascending and descending are the levers of the exiting of Yang energy and entering of Yang's storage. Rising and descending are the two handles that cause Yang to go out of storage or "exit" and back into storage or "enter." These two planes, east-west and north-south, are called Jing and Wei. The north-south plane, or Jing, connects heaven and earth and is where water and fire unite to create life. The east-west plane, or Wei, is where the two levers of ascending and descending give us the motions of life.

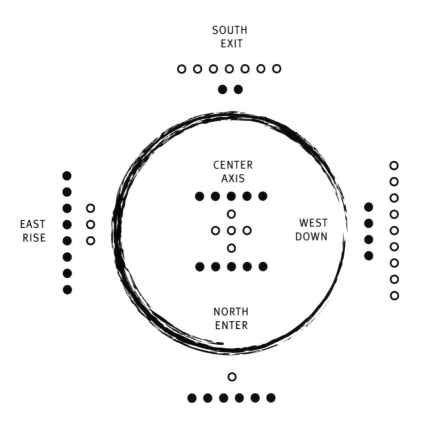

This plane causes the Yang to exit and enter, to expand and contract with every breath we take, on every daily cycle, on every month, and on every year. Every cycle of life's energy is pulled and pushed by the east-west levers.

The Yellow Emperor says that Qi has four directions: rising, descending, exiting, and entering. The River Chart below depicts the attachment of the five Yin organs to the five directions.

The liver, which belongs to the east, is on the left. The lungs, which belong to the west, are on the right. The heart, which belongs to the south, is on the "exiting" and the kidneys, which belong to the north, are on the "entering." The liver and lungs are on the east-west axis, while the heart and kidneys are on the

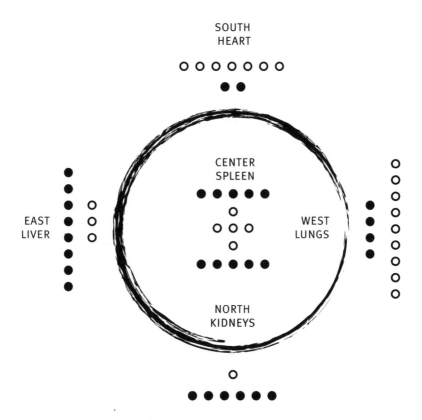

north-south axis. The Yellow Emperor says that the heaven One, which is the heart, descends into the north to create water. He also says that the earth Two, which are the two kidneys, ascend to the south to create fire. This is the reason that we have two kidneys. At the same time, secondary but not less important, are the heaven Three that create wood in the east (or left) and the earth Four that create metal in the west (or right). This is the east-west axis that ensures life is cycling after the initial creation. The heaven Three is an odd number and is why there is one liver, while the earth Four is an even number and why we have two lungs. Finally, we have the number Five, which creates the earth and the spleen. This is the center axis for the Jing and the Wei, as it is likewise the center point for the east-west and north-south axis. As in a revolving wheel, the center of the wheel is the focal point. It has to fix the axis so that the wheel can rotate smoothly without jumping in disarray. The spleen, which is the only organ in the center of the body, has a harmonizing function of all four directions. It is the focal point for the axis.

While the east-west axis is the action during life itself, the north-south axis is the creation and end of life. The heart and the kidneys, or what we previously described as the Shao Yin, is the axis for the creation and end of life — it is the axis for the "entering" and "exiting" of life. When the Yellow Emperor described the heart as distributing to the exterior and the kidneys ruling the interior, it corresponds to this description of the "entering" and "exiting" axis.

Now, let's return to the story of the man who lived his life to its fullest. On his deathbed, he desired only water and to spend time in the warming sun. He felt no desire for food, clothes, or entertainment. Water and sun make up the north-south axis, the origin of life, which unites with death on the same axis. We enter and exit life from the same axis, which connects heaven and earth, water and fire, and Yin and Yang. The heaven One gives birth to water and the earth Two gives birth to fire. The heart warms up the kidneys and the kidneys cool off the heart. One cannot do without the other.

This basic north-south axis requirement for life is the same for fertility and pregnancy. Pregnancy needs the north-south axis. It needs the one and the two, the male and the female. The One and Two start from the male and female hearts as represented by their emotions — love, passion, and desire, and ends with the male and female kidneys represented by their genitalia and reproductive organs. These are a must for a healthy pregnancy and healthy future generations.

The ten months of pregnancy take place in the center of the female body. This is where Yin and Yang are in their most advanced state of harmony, at the spleen pivot point of the two axes. The north-south and east-west cross through the center, and it is because of the center that the north-south axis can transform into the east-west. The primordial life creation (pregnancy) can turn into life itself (baby).

There is a very specific reason why nature designed a man and a woman, a One and a Two, and brought them together. It was to enable the creation of this north-south axis, which during a pregnancy, passes through nine stages, or months, of pregnancy that corresponds to the entire transformation of the "River Chart." Again, the transformations of the "River Chart" are Heaven One gives birth to water and Earth Six completes it. Earth Two gives birth to fire and Heaven Seven completes it. Heaven Three gives birth to wood and Earth Eight completes it. When the entire cycle is complete at the number ten, the fetus can exit the mother with its own east-west axis. It will go back to the north-south axis before death. When conception occurs, the mother and father are horizontal in the east-west axis, but immediately thereafter they stand up and go back to the north-south axis, which is heaven and earth. The fetus is initially horizontal and as the months go by turns into the vertical axis south-north with the head pointing down, but emerging, turns so the head can be pointing upward to heaven.

The baby will still spend the first few months of his life in a horizontal position, crawling until he matures to the point where he can maintain his own north-south axis, when he can sit, stand up, and walk. He will then return to the east-west axis every night when going to sleep. This changing of axis from east-west to north-south is instrumental when it comes to ensuring the prosperity of future generations.

I have questioned a midwife for statistics regarding women who begin labor at night. She estimated that 80 percent of pregnant women go into labor between 11 P.M. and 3 A.M., the time of the Shao Yin. It is the time of the day where the north-south axis is dominant. I asked an oncologist about similar statistics for terminally ill cancer patients, and was told that approximately 70 percent expire at the same Shao Yin time. It is statistically significant that 70 percent of the people die in 17 percent of the day.

During nine months of pregnancy and the tenth month of delivery, a fetus will develop its physical body as it proceeds through creation. During the different stages, different body parts and organs are created and different aspects of the energy and spirit form. Chen Xiuyuan writes in his work *Superficial Comments on the Yellow Emperor*: "This is because the heaven's Qi penetrates through the body and because the body's Qi penetrates through the heavens." The reason that the fetus develops is not because it is a "coincidence." It is because it is influenced by heaven's Qi, or by the life force around us. This is what gives us life. This is what causes our development inside the womb and outside of it.

For all of this to work properly we need a healthy One and Two. We need a healthy man and woman for a perfect north-south axis. The baby will enter the world with an east-west axis and live his life to the fullest until going back to the north-south during the exit.

When the Yellow Emperor says that "the heart distributes to the exterior and the kidneys control the interior," this refers to the "entry" and "exit" of life. The kidneys are used for reproduction and they are the tools for "entry," while the heart is used to connect the spirit to heaven and it is the tool used for "exit." *The Yellow Emperor* says that the five Yin organs transmit their essence to the heart and that the heart connects to the five heaven energies via the eyes. On his deathbed, the old man closes his eyes and this connection between the Yin organs and the heaven's energies subsides. The connection to heaven becomes looser and looser.

When one tries to alter the north-south or east-west with artificial medications and procedures, it is going against nature's intention and is bound to fail. I believe in the old adage: "If you mess with nature, it will mess with you." If you are not in good health and your kidneys are weak at the time of conception, the north-south will not meet, and infertility will result. On the other hand, if you are healthy according to Chinese medicine, your kidneys are strong and your north-south can meet, you are fertile and can become pregnant, whether or not Western medicine has diagnosed you as infertile.

When the parents are healthy in the "north-south fashion" they should trust that the pregnancy they achieved is real. Most intervention in the shape of pills and foreign substances impacting the mother will offset this balance.

QUESTION "THE PILL"

A woman's health and fertility should not be decided by a male-dominated health insurance industry, nor be decided by a pharmaceutical industry heavily influenced by associations with Western medicine. The decision about a woman's fertility should be given to the woman who is seeking the treatment.

Let's take the female menstrual cycle, for example. In my practice, I have seen thousands of patients who have taken the birth control pill for different reasons. Of the patients who had irregular periods before taking the pill, and became regular while on the pill, none of them retained the regularity once discontinuing the pill. Of the patients who had regular periods before taking the pill, and regular periods while on the pill, quite a number became irregular when discontinuing the pill.

In Chinese medicine, we seek harmony with nature and with the lunar cycles when we attempt to regulate the menses. I have witnessed many patients who regulated their periods while taking herbs and Chinese medicine. Not only did their period become regular, it also stayed regular for years after stopping the herbal consumption. In addition, treating infertility with herbs aims at restoring harmony. The goal is to ovulate one egg per lunar cycle, not thirty eggs, which is the goal of modern drugs.

Estrogen and progesterone that occur naturally in the body to regulate the menses is the body's response to the lunar cycles in nature. This cycle will be changed after conception and during pregnancy. The progesterone will not decline but rather increase to maintain the pregnancy. Even though these hormones are physical chemicals, they are not the cause for the menstrual cycle, but are rather a response to the growth and decline of Yin energy.

When a patient who is irregular begins menstruating like clockwork on taking the pill, it is clear that the blood deficiency is still there and even aggravates with time. The drugs may be prompting the menstruation bleeding to happen regularly, but the blood is not strong. This will desynchronize the woman farther from a lunar cycle harmony. In other words, not only is she losing blood every month, the blood is deficient. From the Chinese medicine science perspective, this is not possible according to nature. It is unnatural and in fact is considered "miraculous."

THE MALE ENERGY – NOT AS QUICK AS IT LOOKS

The man participates in the process of creation for approximately two minutes. After that, the woman does it by herself. However, if we can briefly peek into a different dimension—a dimension of spirituality—then the scenario is completely different.

In Chinese medicine, as in many religions, the spirit is an integral part of the body. In Judaism, for example, the body and spirit are analogized as a candle and its flame. The candle is a cup or a vessel holding olive oil, and when it is lit, the flame feeds on the olive oil. The flame cannot exist without the vessel, and although the vessel can exist without the flame, it is just a useless cup. So is the case with our body and spirituality. The body is like the vessel and the spirituality is like the flame. The primary element in our existence here on earth is our spirituality, but we cannot be spiritual without our body and our health.

The two most obvious phenomena we can see in nature are the sun and the moon. In Judaism and in Chinese medicine, the sun is male, constantly radiating hot energy, and the moon is female, receiving the sun's warmth.

While we are warmed and sustained by the outermost layer of the sun, the inside essence of the sun must be transmitted to us in order to create life. To do this, nature created the moon to reflect the sun's inner energy back to us without reflecting its intense heat. This reflection of the essence is the moon's job, but the essence itself is the sun's essence.

The reason that we have a sun and a moon, a male and a female, a Yin and a Yang, is to enable the Yang essence to find a place in the Yin. The sun's essence can be reflected into the moon and then onto earth. The male's essence can be deposited in the female and reflected into the baby. According to the Jewish Kabala, the life's energy begins from above the male, travels into his brain, down his spine, into his kidneys and out through his penis into the female, depositing this sun's essence into the moon to create new life. The new life has started from the sun's essence, or in other words, has been spawned from the male's spirituality.

Again, if we only think in physical terms, then the sperm is just a piece of material produced in the male's testes. The only difference between sperm and a rock is that the sperm has a genetic code on it and the genetic code makes life.

In my view, the modern scientific idea that human genes alone contain the code of life is so superficial and redundant that it is difficult to understand how it is so widely accepted. Simply consider that a sperm, which is microscopic, creates an embryo, fetus, baby, toddler, adult, and an old man or woman—a one-hundred-year cycle of emotions, physical, and spiritual worlds. A sperm must be more than just a microscopic piece of matter. It is similar, in fact, to a nuclear reactor in terms of the power imbedded within.

The sperm is the Yang energy that gives life. It is spiritually powerful. It is transferring the power that resides in the male's health and in his spiritual clearance into the child to come. If the husband's spirit is down, depleted or disturbed, conception cannot happen. This is why so many IVFs fail, because it is difficult to unite the husband's spirit with his sperm in a laboratory. There is no romance or intimacy or love involved. Love, in fact, is spirituality. It is the vehicle, which takes the husband's spirituality into the sperm. A woman becoming pregnant without a loving husband is like the moon existing without the sun.

As *The Great Treatise of Yin and Yang Reflections* states, "Yin and Yang are the paths of heaven and earth, it is the reason for everything on earth, it is the mother and father of transformation, it is the root of birth and decline, it is the palace of the clear spirit."

The palace of the clear spirit and the root of birth are closely related. Clear spirituality provides the optimum conditions for birth. Of course, both parents must be of clear spirit, but the father must develop his spirituality specifically for the purpose of conception, and nurture it from the day he is born until the day he conceives. By contrast, the mother's spirituality is of great importance from the time of conception until the moment she gives birth. After birth, the spirits of both parents unite in an effort to grow the spirituality of their child so that he or she can bear children when the time is right.

The female can take the male essence and make a new life out of it. She takes the light of the male and transforms it into a new kind of light she reflects forward, transforming the previous generation into a new one.

Chinese medicine theory is so developed that most people simply can't understand it today and modern science lags far behind it. Nevertheless, some bright Western scientists are looking beyond the normal quota. For example, Dr. Johanna Budwig, a seven-time Nobel Prize nominee, writes in her book *Flax Oil as Aid against Cancer*, "The living mass of mankind derives its being, as does all life in nature, from the sun! This has been forgotten until now in biology and medical science." She also writes, "Solar energy electrons are both wave and matter!"

Nobel winner Louis De Broglie wrote that "light is the fastest, purest, lightest and most beautiful form of matter we know, as well as the fastest and purest form of energy we are aware of. As the fast emissary from star to star, sunlight electrons are always, whatever their condition, both wave and matter. The electron is a form of matter always surrounded by magnetism. It can be measured as either matter or wave. This borderline situation between energy and matter overturns all classical physics, and is extraordinarily interesting as well as of vital importance in respect of physiological, medical and biological problems."

What is "energy and matter" if not the concept of heaven and earth, and Yin and Yang? The next step in modern science development will be the improvement of Western medicine into a different realm, from a physical world into an "energy and life force" world. This will then become closer to the Chinese medicine realm.

MALE VITALITY – ALL YOU NEED IS LOVE

The "thought" that is the seed of conception descends from the male brain, down his spine, to his kidneys and out his penis as a white drop ready to enter into his female partner. The penis is like a dead organ. Ninety-nine percent of the time it is shrunken and useless. For a brief moment every day, or every week or every month, the penis becomes alive due to the "thought." The testicles are simply the home of the physical sperm, the sperm's energy emanating from the "thought" and from the spirit.

Many men are devastated by the infertility treatments administered to their wives. Physically, the sperm seems to be fine. All the drugs, laparoscopes, and procedures are aimed at the prospective mother. The husband, longing to impregnate his wife, has an inborn need to imbue the next life in the woman just like the sun gives its essence to the moon. He also has the innate impulse to protect his wife from harm at a time when infertility treatments are placing her in harm's way due to side effects, surgery, pain and financial stress. This situation creates havoc in the male's spirit. It is nearly impossible for him to transfer his spirituality into the sperm, and hence, it is nearly impossible for the wife to become pregnant.

In a couple's relationship and desire for a baby, the male's spirituality is key. The vitality of his spirit is just as or more important than the vitality of his physical body. In the past, women were considered inferior to men. Although this has thankfully changed today, the new dynamic that men and women are equal has spawned a new assumption that no matter what happens, the male will never feel inferior, emasculated, and spiritually broken. This is a big mistake. Many men have a broken spirit because of this new dynamic. You can't see it from the outside, but the problem is there.

The solution is love, for that alone is what will make the dynamic work. Love means that the wife feels she will do whatever her husband wants, and in turn the husband feels that he will do whatever his wife wants. No husband wants to see his wife get hurt and no wife wants to see her husband emasculated. The woman makes the man happy by keeping his male vitality intact. She does this by vibrating a message to him that communicates that she loves him and he is enough. This in turn allows him to protect and provide for his wife, the true joy of the husband.

The wife does not rely entirely on her spirituality to nourish the fetus. She rather relies on her Yin energy, as well as her blood. When the wife's Yin spirit and blood suffer, the couple can still become pregnant, but it is highly likely that there will be a miscarriage.

In my practice, both partners receive herbal treatment, although the wife does receive more of the treatment as she does with Western procedures. The difference is that with my treatment, the husband knows that his wife is growing healthier, and hence, he has the ability to protect his wife, and his vitality is not compromised.

THE ESSENCE OF SPIRITUALITY

The sun, as far as we know, is a great ball of fire. Yet it is different than the fire in your kitchen, which must be cautiously fed in order to keep itself going. The sun, on the other hand, is eternal. Its flame runs on a different source: the internal essence of the sun.

The sun reflects in us as human beings and especially in men. It keeps us running with its eternal essence. In Judaism, Christianity, Buddhism, Daoism, and all other religions, this essence is virtue —the will power to do good deeds, charity, and other beneficial actions for others. It is what makes us want to love our child or help a friend.

This virtue is the spirituality source of life. Although women have virtue too, virtue is the male's strongest quality. This is the same source that feeds down to the male brain and "thought," down the spine, the kidneys, and out the penis into the female partner.

The moon receives the essence of the sun, becomes pregnant with it, and then reflects it to women on earth. This energy is about bravery. Because the moon predominantly impacts the woman, the woman's strongest quality is courage and strength. When a woman becomes pregnant and delivers a baby, her courage is beyond anything a man can imagine.

When a man deposits his virtue through his white drop (semen and sperm), the woman possesses the courage to harbor it, and becomes pregnant with it. The courage continues by the internal source of the moon. Every month the moon disappears, but then has the courage to come back for another cycle. The woman will find the courage in her to become pregnant and deliver a baby, to raise the child through difficult times and hardship. Without the courage of the woman, there would be no life.

The virtue quality that men possess is also about "letting go." He lets go of his sperm—and the necessary accompanying spirit—when he releases it into the woman. The courage of a woman is embodied in "holding on," even clinging to things. This spirit is needed for holding on to the sperm and onto pregnancy. This energy is also needed for building a home for the family.

Both men and women need courage and virtue throughout their lives, but when a man has too much courage, or when a woman has too much virtue, problems may result. It is the same as relying on the moon to warm us, or the sun to reflect on us. The sun, although warming and lighting the way during the day, cannot dispel the darkness at night as the moon can. The sun is simply absent altogether at night. It does not have the brave quality that the moon exhibits.

Dan suffered from erectile dysfunction, which only occurred around his wife's ovulation. Dan's doctor recommended Viagra. Nevertheless, Dan and his wife did not conceive for three years, even with two IVF cycles. Dan came to me and received herbal treatment and within three months the erectile function recovered and within two months the couple conceived. His problem was a deteriorated heart fire aggravated by "trying to conceive" pressure. He improved to the point that his wife no longer needed to chart temperature or use ovulation kits. Dan says that it was much easier without all the pressure.

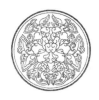

.....4.....

UNDERSTANDING INFERTILITY
THE RIGHT WAY

THE LIFE INSIDE YOUR WOMB

"Goodness-of-fit" is a child psychology term first used by Thomas and Chess in 1977. It explains that the social environment of a child will impact the child's future development. A mother has certain expectations from her child even from before it is born. She doesn't want her child to be sick or misbehave. She does want her child to be healthy, strong, and intelligent. When a child behaves the way his mother wishes, it is referred to as a "goodness-of-fit."

It is the same case in the reverse role. A child has certain expectations of his mother. He wants her to be nourishing, warm, and understanding of his frustrations. He does not want his mother to abandon him, ignore him, or shout at him. When a mother behaves in a way that fulfills the child's wishes, it is "goodness-of-fit."

Thomas and Chess explain that "goodness-of-fit" allows the child to develop in a positive way—to grow into a fulfilled adult. Without it, the child will no doubt have emotional issues as an adult.

This "goodness-of-fit" is just as important in the womb as it is outside. In Western medicine, the most important priority to ensure that fit is making certain the baby is receiving the proper vitamins. But the baby needs much more than that. The baby needs a lifeline. Where there is no life to carry, the child cannot be born.

THE SIX SPHERES OF ENERGY

To understand lifeline we must first be very clear about the significance of Yin and Yang. The six spheres include three Yin and three Yang, both sides comprised of opening, closing, and pivot. To understand the difference between the three Yang and the three Yin, it is helpful to put things into the concept of "time." As we have seen in previous chapters, each of the six spheres has a different time during a Yin and Yang full twenty-four-hour, 29.5 day, or twelve-month cycle.

For simplification purposes, I will only use a twenty-four-hour day cycle and A, B, C instead of the Chinese names of the time periods. First, let's review the locations of the time periods during the day.

Each time period extends two hours in length, giving us a total of twelve time periods within one twenty-four-hour period. Segment "A" is from 11 P.M. to 1 A.M., "B" is from 1 A.M. to 3 A.M., "C" is from 3 A.M. to 5 A.M. and so forth.

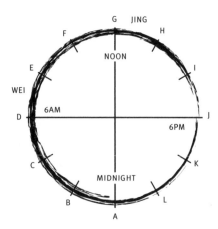

The Tai Yang phase starts from "A" and finishes at "G." "A," around midnight, is the time where the new Yang energy is the coldest, having just been born. "G," around noon, is when the Yang energy is opened up the widest at the warmest time of the day. Yang Ming starts at "G" (noon), the Yang slowly closing down until it reaches its most closed state at "A," or midnight.

This "opening" and "closing" process requires a pivot, the Shao Yang minister fire. The more the Yang energy opens, the higher goes the temperature—whether that corresponds to the time of day, or the seasons of the year. To open, the Tai Yang needs the help of the minister fire.

While Tai Yang needs to be close to the minister fire, the Yang Ming needs to distance itself from the fire in order to close. Consequently, Zhongjing explains in the *Shang Hanlun* that the Shao Yang minister fire time is in the east from "C" until "E", while the Yang Ming time is exactly opposite, from "I" until "K" in the west. The Shao Yang minister fire helps warm up the Tai Yang because it is overlapping the same time period, and also helps cool off the Yang Ming because it is far away from the Yang Ming or opposite to it. This is the "pivot" function of the three Yang spheres.

If the three Yang spheres—opening, closing and pivot—occupy the entire twenty-four hours of the day, where do the three Yin

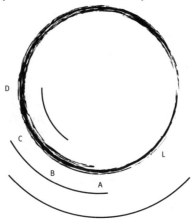

spheres fit in? According to Zhang Zhongjing's description in the *Shang Hanlun*, the Tai Yin sphere begins at "L" and continues to "B." Shao Yin is from "A" until "C," while Jue Yin is from "B" to "D."

The three Yin occupy a much shorter time period than the Yang, from 9 p.m. until 7 a.m. The Yin and Yang, then, are not equal in quantity.

The Yellow Emperor classics explain in great detail the three Yin and three Yang. Each one of the six spheres has a root energy and a manifestation, which was explained in chapter two. These are the Tai Yang cold water, Shao Yang minister fire, Yang Ming dry metal, Tai Yin damp earth, Shao Yin emperor fire and Jue Yin wind wood.

Within the three Yin, Tai Yin is "opening," Jue Yin is "closing," and Shao Yin is the "pivot." From a superficial point of view it seems that "opening," "closing." and "pivot" is quite easy to understand. The Yin opens up, the Yin closes down, and there is a pivot that helps harmonize their opening and closing. In reality, this is not so. It is not like a simple machine.

Observe the four seasons. In three of the four—spring, summer, and fall—we are able to watch the state of the Yang energy with our naked eye (leaves budding, flourishing and falling). However, in winter we cannot see the Yang energy in storage (trees are naked). We can, however, sense it with our heart.

This same phase is the storage phase that Zhongjing attributes

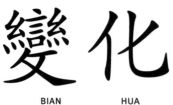

BIAN　　　　HUA

to the Yin spheres—the time of darkness. So why do we have Yin altogether? We need to look back to the Chinese medicine classics to understand. The Yellow Emperor describes the annual four seasons in five phases, including the birth and growth phases representing the spring and summer, and the wood and fire elements respectively. Then there is a transformation phase, "Hua," which represents the late summer and the earth element. Following "transformation" are the decline and storage phases representing the fall and winter, and metal and water elements respectively.

The Yang commences opening at midnight and stops opening at noon, when there is transformation allowing the Yang to return into storage to become stronger. If the Yang energy goes into storage and does not reemerge, this is death. The Yellow Emperor then omits the word from the sequence. He does not insert "death" between the winter's storage and the spring's birth. Here, where the word "Bian" was supposed to be, we are allowed to enter the realm of the three Yin, from where the Yang re-springs the next morning. The reason we are able to wake up every morning is the three Yin, which are the root of life.

Our next step is to understand what actually happens in the three Yin that propels our life forward, and why the Shao Yin emperor fire serves as an axis.

For this purpose, we turn to several quotes from the classic *Miraculous Pivot*—Chapter of Ying and Wei. This classic often refers to Shao Yin and Yang Ming as the core of Yin and Yang and in this chapter it also mentions the function of the Tai Yin and Tai Yang. It says: "The man receives his energy (Qi) from the food, the food enters the stomach and then the energy is transported to the lungs, then the five Yin and six Yang organs all receive energy."

From this ancient text we can see the function of the three Yang and some of the function of the three Yin. When water and food enter our stomach, they are transformed into our Yang energy. This Yang energy takes many shapes and forms. It can be the energy of the inner organs, it can become the protective energy that defends us from harmful influences or it can also be the nutritive energy that nourishes our body. The Yellow Emperor describes this energy as reaching the "four seas," meaning every aspect of our life.

The ancient text explains: "When Yang energy reaches the Yang phase it starts moving and when it reaches the Yin phase it stops."

Knowing that our energy circulates fifty times in our body during one day and one night, the ancients explained that the Yang stops "fifty cycles and the energy returns to Da Hui (big meeting place)." Da Hui means at midnight or at the time of A – 11 P.M.– 1:00 A.M. The text then explains that at midnight, where Da Hui happens, all the people are asleep. Midnight is the time where all the Yang energy returns. This is the time when the three Yin take action.

When we talk about the Yin and Yang energies in our body, they are not heaven and earth but rather water and fire. The Yin of our body is coming from the three Yin of heaven (Kan – water) and the Yang of our body is coming from the three Yang of heaven (Li – fire). What we get from the earth is our body. When a person dies, even though the Yang energy separates from the Yin energy and both are extinct, the body of the person is still lying on the ground lifeless. The dead body does not have any Yang energy or any Yin energy. It belongs to the earth. It has no Xing or Ming. The energy of the body—three Yin and three Yang—belongs to heaven.

INFERTILITY AND SHAO YIN – ESSENCES EXCHANGED

Our life relies on "true fire," which belongs to the same category as the Yang energy, yet it is not the same as Yang energy. "True fire" is the Shao Yin emperor fire. In the Shao Yin there are two organs, heart and kidneys. The heart represents fire and it is the emperor organ in the Chinese medicine anatomy, while the kidneys represent water and are responsible for reproduction and the sex organs. Heart and kidneys compose the post-heaven water-fire relationship needed for life.

In *The Book of Changes*, Yi Jing, states that "The male and female exchange essences and then the myriad things are born." What is the meaning of this quote? Fire is the man's desire, which stems from the heart, for the woman and the woman's desire for the man. Water is the reliance on the sex organs for sexual activity and reproduction. The exchange of water and fire is necessary for the exchange of male and female essences. When the water or fire is deficient, the exchange cannot be complete. If the exchange of essences is not complete, then the likelihood of a pregnancy is decreased. This is what we call infertility.

In modern medicine, all research is focused on Xing, the material, and nothing is focused on Ming, the lifeline energy. This is why patients and doctors alike are occupied with physical findings such as hormones, fibroids, cysts, and fallopian tubes, as if something "physical" must be obstructing the conception's "physical" process.

In reality this is not the case. The main cause of infertility is an obstacle with the "lifeline." The essences of the fire and water from the father and/or mother have a problem. This is why many of my male patients have "perfect" sperm, but cannot conceive with their wives until their Shao Yin is brought into balance. This is also the case with many of my female patients who suffer "unexplained" or "explained" infertility and yet, when their Shao Yin true fire is fixed, they can get pregnant.

We can see that the clear and most purified energy derived from our food, water, and the air we breathe, enters into the Yin spheres to help with the emperor fire's activity of "saving life." The father and mother have Shao Yin water-fire activity. The embryo needs it as well. If the father and mother are lacking the essences of water and fire, then the embryo cannot form. Treating infertility is the treatment of water and fire. It is the treatment of Shao Yin. After seeing many patients, I can testify that at least seven or eight out of every ten have a Shao Yin problem, with symptoms such as cold hands and feet, hot flashes followed by a cold feeling, slightly red face with a thirst for warm liquids, thin and small pulse, and exhaustion as a result of insomnia. I normally use herbal formulas to strengthen the Shao Yin water and fire, and many of my patients are blessed with beautiful babies.

THE CONSTANT LINK

Shao Yin disease, then, is the main cause of infertility. This statement seems simple but in reality has many variables. Many religions explain that when we die, our bodies return to earth, and our spirits return to heaven. However, from one generation to the other, there is a continuous link. It is not only heaven and earth that we need, but rather the direct lifeline from our parents. If this lifeline is broken, life stops.

As we explained above, there is Ming—pre-heaven—and there is Xing, which is post-heaven. Diseases can arise in either of these states. In our daily life (Xing) we can do the wrong things that will make us sick; in our embryonic life (Ming) our parents can do the wrong things that will make us sick or shorten our life. The cervical cancer cases from DES, for example, represent a pre-heaven disease, in that they were a direct result of actions taken by the mother. Even though most of us want to do the right things when we are pregnant so our baby will be healthy, we may have a serious problem fulfilling that wish because we are relying solely on the knowledge of modern science. Medical doctors are occupied with the prevention of immediate birth defects; however, defects beyond birth are no less important. How will the baby grow up to be an adult? How will he or she reproduce and create another generation? These questions are completely outside the scope of Western medicine. In contrast, Chinese medicine has researched the long-term effects of treatment, passing the knowledge down from one generation to the next.

MEDICINE IS IN THE DOCTOR'S HEART

"Yi Zhe Xin Ye" is an ancient Chinese idiom that means "medicine is heart." Chen Xiuyuan in his book, *Prescriptions Poems from Chang Sha*, wrote: "The good or bad fortune of the patient is entrusted to the doctor. Thus the doctor's responsibility is great. However, the power is not entrusted in the hand of medicine, but rather in the hand of the person practicing the medicine."

The natural desire to assist another person in need was designated by Confucius as "virtue." The desire to help the sick was designated by the sage as Yi De meaning "medicine's virtue," which all who learn to practice medicine must have. A sick person is defined as anyone who has lost his or her balance, either within himself or with his surroundings. Whether it is Yin or Yang, the doctor's responsibility is to know the origin of the problem, which medicinal remedy to use for treatment, and how to bring this patient back to harmony. The reason behind studying medicine and becoming a doctor, according to the sages, is only one: to help sick people become healthier. If the doctor follows this path of virtue he becomes one with the Dao. He is a true doctor.

The doctor's virtue pushes him on an endless quest for knowledge. He wants to know how to ensure the safety and health of his patients. When a doctor adopts a path that causes his patient's health to deteriorate, even if he is not aware of it, the offense under heaven is unparalleled. With heavy weight on their shoulders, the sages put their lives at stake in the quest for truth in medicine. When and if the physician made a mistake at the imperial court, he would lose his head the next day.

Today, many doctors in Western and Chinese medicine save lives on a daily basis and their work is unmatched. On the other hand, many others ruin lives. The difference lies in their possession or absence of virtue.

For example, a patient who recently underwent IVF began the drug protocol perfectly healthy and with no complaints. Within a few days of ingesting the drugs, her tongue coating began to deteriorate, and a week later, the rear half of the tongue coating was completely missing. She suddenly began feeling weak and tired, and the skin over the front of her leg became sensitive as if there were needles underneath it.

I treated the patient with acupuncture, but this could not save her kidney's essence, nor could it help her original Yang. I felt as if an invisible hand entered my heart and squeezed it. The pain stayed with me until the evening. When she asked her doctor about these "side effects" he plainly dismissed them as "normal."

The situation is not as grave with modern Chinese medicine; however, it has similarities. Patients with deficient original Yang are often diagnosed as Yin deficient and receive greasy, thick, cold herbs harming their lifeline further.

The job of the patient is to educate herself and tune herself into her condition. If she believes her condition is worsening with treatment, she must transition to another option.

IVF AND THE ROOT OF LIFE

As we now understand the importance of a lifeline, I want to share with you my personal Chinese medicine experience with IVF and fertility drugs. During an IVF treatment, heavy doses of various synthetic drugs and synthetic hormones are utilized. Patients typically suffer side effects, such as feeling hot flashes followed by immediately feeling cold, a bloated lower abdomen, irregular periods, headaches, lower back pain, red tongue, slow pulse, as well as the deterioration of the tongue coating to patchy or completely missing.

From a classical Chinese medicine point of view, these symptoms are all under the same category of deteriorating Shao Yin and diminishing "true fire."

The Yellow Emperor says, "The core principle of Yin and Yang is that the Yang condenses and then the Yin becomes resolute." This means that when Yang can condense inward, Yin can begin performing its three steps of preserving life as we discussed previously: prepare the earth, add true fire to create damp/mist, and quickly finish the process of the first two. When a patient uses fertility drugs and hormone therapy, according to Chinese medicine thinking, either the three Yang are harmed (feeling cold or tired) or the three Yin are damaged (hot flashes, bloated abdomen, clouded spirit). Yang energy is unable to condense and Yin energy cannot be resolute.

Under normal circumstances, a woman is able to discharge one egg per menstrual cycle. How then, while using fertility drugs and hormones, is she able to discharge twenty or thirty eggs? According to Chinese medicine principles, this excessive extraction of "true fire" is able to sever the root of life, and any such severing can last for several generations. For example, studies many years after WWII have shown that the stress resulting from widespread famine in Holland during the War caused impairment in genes for at least two successive generations.

With aggressive fertility treatment, when the father's or mother's heart fire and kidney water are damaged by drugs and synthetic hormones, what will the consequences be for their children and grandchildren? It is unclear at this point, and I cannot pretend to predict the future. However, Chinese medicine explains that we must do our best to preserve the lifeline we hand down to our children. This lifeline is all within the Shao Yin water and fire essences we exchange with our husband or wife. In Chinese medicine, we say that the most important element when treating a disease is to correctly differentiate the syndrome before treating it. We differentiate and treat for one reason: to preserve the root of life.

Let us think about it from a logical point of view. In your opinion, if you are ill and you become pregnant, could that impact your child's future? We can't give a definite answer. It might not impact your child. But let us reverse the question and ask: if you are very healthy, on a honeymoon or vacation, and feel great while you conceive, could that be beneficial for your baby? It will not hurt and probably will be beneficial. When we undergo excessive drug therapy, or for that matter any kind of therapy, and suffer "side effects," does that mean we are healthy or not healthy? In conventional medicine, where the disease is the target and not the person, we are taught that "side effects" are known to the drug manufacturer and thus, we should learn how to "live with it." But from the Chinese medicine point of view, there is nothing "side" about "side effects." For example, if a woman undergoing IVF begins to experience hot flashes, one mechanism in the body is out of order and disharmony and illness symptoms result. Although it is difficult to prove that this will harm the baby, because it would be necessary to follow the study for several generations, we can use logic to assume that it may.

Another point that must be considered when we discuss IVF is the low success rate. Why is there only a 5 percent success rate for patients older then forty-two? Modern medicine claims poor egg quality. In reality, the situation is quite different. As we age, the original Yang declines until it is consumed completely when we die. A forty-year-old patient has less original Yang than a twenty-year-old. When using fertility drugs, where the original Yang is undergoing heavy extraction in order to produce more eggs, the forty-year-old patient is exhausted beyond her "true fire" reserves. Three days later, when the woman undergoes an embryo transfer, it cannot be supported by true fire because there is none left. This is why nineteen out of twenty patients fail. However, when using donor eggs, the success rate rises again because the donor egg is much younger, or so assumes modern medicine.

My experience shows differently. In a donor egg cycle, the patient is not stimulated, and thus her true fire is not exhausted. It is the donor woman who is losing her true fire during stimulation. So the forty-year-old patient receives an embryo while she still has some true fire left. I am certain that one hundred years from now, Western doctors will look back at the procedures and drugs used today and view them as archaic. I will not be surprised if Chinese medicine herbs and theory will occupy a bigger role.

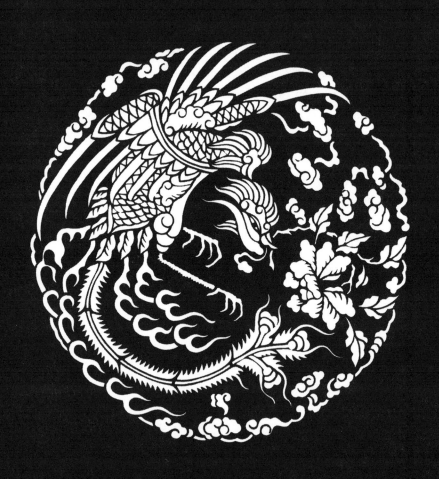

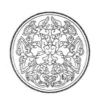

····5····

FERTILITY OBSTACLES

By presenting several patient accounts and threading them together, I want to share with you my view from the practitioner's side about what I believe are the major obstacles to achieving fertility.

DRUG CRAZY

Abigail (all names are fictitious), a twenty-seven-year-old female, discontinued birth control pills approximately a year ago after using them for ten years. Since stopping her use of the pill, her menstruation has stopped. A reproductive endocrinologist induced a period by giving her more fertility drugs and estrogen and progesterone treatments. While using the fertility drugs, she produced more than twenty follicles and was told she no longer met the qualifications for IUI (artificial insemination). The RE recommended in vitro fertilization (IVF). His diagnosis for Abigail's condition was that "the patient is very athletic and thinly built, which is causing her absent periods." When asked about her weight, Abigail explained to me that she gained ten pounds in the past year. According to my calculation, her weight is normal for her height and build. She agreed with her RE and started an IVF cycle. She was eager to get pregnant with the help of the drugs and stated, "I don't want to waste any more time."

Lisa is a forty-five-year-old female who underwent seven IUI procedures and six IVF procedures within a two-year period. Each procedure failed. After using the Hunyuan herbal treatment for two months, she conceived naturally. After conception, Lisa expressed concern about consuming herbs during her pregnancy, and discontinued use. She returned to her doctor and began receiving progesterone shots. A miscarriage followed.

Wendy, a thirty-eight-year-old female, underwent three IUIs with Clomid and later with injectable drugs. She reported feeling sick to her stomach with severe night sweats and anxiety attacks. After one month of herbal treatment with the Hunyuan Method, the symptoms subsided. Wendy went back to the doctor who asserted that the dosage had been too weak in the previous cycle, and decided to begin another medicated IUI with twice the dosage. The cycle failed and all the side effects returned stronger than ever.

Joanne is a forty-six-year-old female who suffered secondary infertility, the inability to conceive after having a child. She received Hunyuan herbal treatment and acupuncture for six months. Although she did not conceive, her symptoms of achy joints and arthritis-like pain disappeared during the course of herbal protocols. Returning to IUI with medications, the pain returned within the first ten days. Joanne expressed concern yet commented: "I know the drugs are harmful, but I can always come back so you can fix me up. My plan is to do a few cycles and hopefully I can come out of it fast enough before I am burned out."

CONVENTIONAL DIAGNOSIS BREEDS PSYCHOLOGICAL FAILURE

Sally, a thirty-three-year-old female, conceived naturally but suffered a miscarriage. A Dilation & Curettage (D&C) was done to speed up the cleaning of the uterus lining. The patient could not conceive for a year after the D&C. The Western diagnosis was that she had poor egg quality.

Brenda, a forty-three-year-old female, had secondary infertility. The Western diagnosis was that she was too old to get pregnant. Karina, a thirty-nine-year-old female, failed three IVFs. The Western diagnosis was that she had elevated FSH levels. Madeline is a forty-year-old female who suffered recurrent miscarriages. The Western diagnosis was that she had genetic abnormalities. Terri is a thirty-seven-year-old female who cannot get pregnant. The Western diagnosis was unexplained infertility.

Is there a negative impact on a woman when she is told by an authoritative doctor that her eggs are too old? Or that she is unexplainably infertile? I have seen many patients, who, when told that their eggs are too old, have broken into tears and fallen into depression for days and even months. On the other hand, I have never seen a patient become depressed when hearing that she had a kidney Yang deficiency.

Why is a Western diagnosis so devastating? Because it has a tone of finality. The patient's mind goes into a state of shock. The more it is believed as truth, the more devastating. The new emotional blockage can in fact induce infertility, which in Chinese medicine is referred to as "diminishing the emperor fire." The belief in one's ability to produce a baby has just diminished. I have seen patients become pregnant simply by restoring their self-belief. Follicle Stimulating Hormone (FSH) levels of fifteen are considered a sign of infertility, yet I have had patients with FSH levels of twenty, thirty, and even as high as eighty who conceived naturally.

The emperor fire is in the heart and the willpower is in the kidneys. When they are both functioning correctly, the Shao Yin sphere is intact and fertility will happen.

MAKING BABIES – IT TAKES TWO

When it comes to conception and making babies, it is a job for two: the husband and wife, another manifestation of Yin and Yang. The two are inseparable. When the Yin is impaired, the Yang is in trouble, and when the Yang is obstructed, the Yin is malnourished. There is no such a thing as the problem of the Yin or the problem of the Yang. It is always the problem of both Yin and Yang. That is very different from modern Western medicine where a diagnosis that pronounces the woman infertile or the man sterile creates a separation of the Yin-Yang bond. It becomes the problem of the wife or the husband, but not both. When the wife is diagnosed with poor egg quality and the husband is celebrated with excellent sperm count, it is a terrible blow to the Yin and Yang bond. Even in modern Chinese medicine, practitioners will pronounce the Yin as deficient but the Yang as fine, and vice versa. However, the Yang cannot be fine if the Yin is deficient, for it means that there is no healthy bond between the two. They are separated.

In Chinese medicine, the emperor fire plays a major role in allowing conception to occur. If the husband's emperor fire is lacking, conception will not happen even if his sperm is viable. I have had experiences where I have boosted the morale of the husband over the course of an hour conversation, and then seen the couple conceive within the month. The wife became much more content during that month, which was enough for her to become pregnant.

THE INTERNET – JUST THE BEGINNING OF KNOWLEDGE

We know that the quest for knowledge is an important one and that the Internet is certainly a significant tool. However, because Chinese medicine is an art that has crystallized over thousands of years, we must be careful how we take the Internet's online information into account.

Online research gives us pieces of information in greater and greater volume but with diminishing quality. While it gives us facts, it does not necessarily provide real knowledge or understanding. In the past, one would have borrowed books from a library, or taken a course on a particular subject. This might have taken days, months, or even years to accomplish. In a world of easy and rapid information disbursement, this search can take only minutes and does not guarantee accurate information. It becomes difficult for us to know whom we should follow and what we should learn.

One cannot get to the essence of Chinese medicine from pieces of information even if it is accurate, let alone if it is wrong. We are far better off relying on the wisdom of the past tested in the laboratory of history.

We must understand science to grasp the heart of the problem. Science is emotionless. Its principle is to find the cold facts and its goal is to replicate the results. If I analyze data scientifically, the results must be reliable. This means that if I analyze similar data later, the results must be the same, otherwise the first results were wrong. This instrument of science is, of course, very useful in many areas, including modern medicine, aviation, and tecȲology.

Yet when we talk about art, the concept is different. When we look at a painting, listen to music, or watch a movie, something happens in the object we see that moves our heart. Art has no cold scientific boundaries. Rather, it has to do with the skill of the artist and the eye of the beholder.

Chinese medicine is an art too. The eyes of the practitioner and the health of the patient are both unique. The skill of the practitioner plays a crucial role. This can be a disadvantage, as some practitioners are less skilled than others. But the skills of the practitioner can also exceed normal levels, allowing his touch to bring a cure. Achieving results are not as simple as duplicating a procedure, which is the case with modern medicine.

This unique position of Chinese medicine brings big promise and responsibility simultaneously. The practitioner must be on a quest to improve his or her skills for an entire lifetime. The more skill and experience brought to bear, the more effective the cures will be.

The patient gathering pieces of information on the Internet is putting herself in a maze that is difficult to maneuver. She must take two steps away from the monitor. It is fine to gather information, but she must know that this is not knowledge that she can safely and effectively put into use. It is just the beginning of knowledge.

Sarah and James could not conceive for four years. Their doctor explained that James's sperm count was low and that the sperm mobility was below normal. Four IUI and two IVF cycles proved fruitless and their frustration grew. The couple heard from a coworker about me and the Hunyuan Method and decided they had nothing to lose. My conclusion was that Sarah had a Shao Yin kidney deficieny. After five months of Sarah taking herbs and undergoing acupuncture treatments, the couple conceived naturally. James was startled and excited after so many years believing that it was solely his problem.

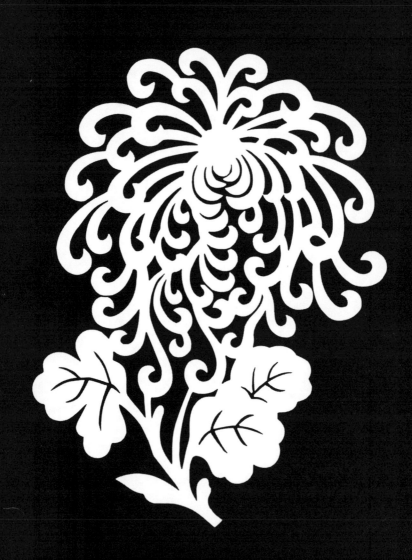

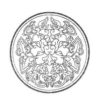

····6····

HERBS, ACUPUNCTURE, AND DIET— DEEPENING UNDERSTANDING

In your quest for fertility, you must first control the spirit. Second, you must know how to nourish the body. Third, you must know the real truth about "toxic" herbs. Fourth, you must understand acupuncture. And fifth, you must know how to understand and diagnose the patterns of the inner organs, the blood, and energy. When you know all of the above, the right path is no longer mysterious.

These are the methods known for the past 3,000 years that bring us closer to health and fertility. We must control the spirit and nourish the body, know herbs and acupuncture, and understand how to diagnose the problem according to Chinese medicine.

THE MIRACLE HERB

The "miracle herb" in Chinese medicine is an herb that performs wonders in your body. If you are very ill, it can make you healthy. If you are sad, it can make you happy. This miracle herb can even give you longevity.

By miracle herbs, we are referring to "Chinese herbs," and there are hundreds of them, each one offering its own specific miracle. There are no single cure-alls. Herbs are Chinese medicine's main tool to restore health and fertility, and combined with acupuncture, they have been the single most practiced and tested healing method for the past 3,000 years.

The challenge is that each single herb must be used exactly at the right time, in the right quantity, and in the right combination with other herbs. It must be prepared correctly, cooked exactly the appropriate length of time, and administered in the correct way. When a patient visits me for the first time and says that she has heard that Dang Gui is good for infertility, I can only politely disagree. The herb is neither good nor bad. If one knows how to use it, it can work miracles. If one doesn't know how to use it effectively, then it is all a matter of chance. As I've stated before, Chinese medicine is not about luck, but rather about knowledge: how to, when to, why to? That is the reason I urge patients to avoid buying herbs for a "quick fix" solution. The patient must be thoroughly versed in the herb, and aware of the long-term effects; that does not mean the results of a study done over a period of six months or two years.

I recently visited a friend in California whose backyard garden is full of medicinal herbs. Every morning he picks a different set of herbs to brew his morning tea. When I looked at him harvesting his herbs, I asked myself: *Is he going to have a long healthy life?* The answer was *absolutely*. Sometimes you look at something and you just know in your heart that it is right. Harvesting his homegrown herbs fresh every morning is in accord with nature. A double blind study is not necessary to prove it true.

Herbal formulas are not made up of a bunch of herbs put together, but rather of ingredients carefully chosen to go into the mix. The practitioner must have adequate knowledge in a variety of areas in order to put an effective formula together. According to an ancient treatise, "When the sages prepared herbs, they had rules for cooking and rules for drinking the herbal teas. Some herbs need to be cooked for a long time, while other herbs cannot be cooked for long. Some herbs require strong flame, while others require low heat for their cooking. These are the main rules of cooking. For drinking, some herbs need to be consumed warm while others cold, some need to be sipped slow while others fast. Some herbs need to be consumed with emotions such as anger or happiness and these emotions help the action of the herbs, while other herbs are contraindicated to emotions. For these contraindicated herbs, the emotions are enemies. These are the rules for drinking the herbs. In addition, some spring water is good and some is bad, so if the patient receives herbs and they don't always work, don't blame the herbs for that. This is because there is difficulty in determining the right way to prepare and drink the herbs."

While establishing the basis for herbal treatments, the Yellow Emperor defines the strategy needed for healing by saying that when the disease is hot, then cool it off, and when the disease is cold, then warm it up. This is the most basic approach for using herbs in classical Chinese medicine. However, the Yellow Emperor does not stop there. In *The Great Treatise of the Five Common Affairs*, he says: "To treat hot disease you use cold herbs and you need to drink it warm. To treat cold disease you use hot herbs and you need to drink it cool. To treat warm disease you use cool herbs and you need to drink it cold. To treat cool disease you use warm herbs and you need to drink it hot." For the herbs to be effective, the method of delivery must be correct.

The book *Stories of Famous Physicians of the Past* includes a story about the famed physician Li Shicai: "One patient suffered cold injury. He felt very agitated and his face was red. His mind was in chaos and at times he wanted to drink cold water. The patient was waving his hands and kicking his feet so that the doctor could not feel his pulse. It took five or six people to subdue the patient for the doctor to take his pulse. The pulse was surging big and without rhythm. When he pressed down on the pulse it felt like a thin thread. Doctor Li said: 'Floating and big, while deep and small it is a Yin disease that looks like a Yang disease. I will give the patient 'strengthening the center decoction' (hot herbs) and he will live.' His student said: 'Ten out of ten doctors would have used cold herbs, but you instead used hot herbs. What is the logic behind it?' Dr. Li answered: 'With warm herbs the patient will live, while with cool herbs he will die. Following this, the doctor decocted the formula 'strengthening the center decoction,' which included four ounces Ginseng and one ounce of Fu Zi. The finished tea was inserted into well water to cool off, and the patient drank it cool. Within one hour the erratic behavior stopped and one cup of tea later, the patient's spirit became clear. With the help of five pounds of herbs, the patient completely recovered."

In this story, we witness the great skill of the physician. The symptoms the patient displayed—red face, waving his hands, etc. —were all hot symptoms, but within the pulse the doctor found the real cause of the disease, a cold disease. Furthermore, in addition to using hot herbs to counter the cold disease, the patient was ordered to cool off the tea before drinking. Doctor Li understood that to bring the hot herbs into the cold disease, the tea must be cool; to bring the south into the north we need the west.

USING HERBS INCORRECTLY THE WESTERN MEDICINE WAY

I customarily treat patients suffering from night sweats and hot flashes with hot herbs. The prevailing reason for night sweats and hot flashes is a deficiency in the Yang energy due to the Yang's inability to root in the kidneys. It is not, as some people believe, a kidney Yin deficiency.

When do women suffer hot flashes most frequently? It is as they approach menopause in their forties and fifties, when the Yang energy is declining for both men and women. If the decline is abnormally rapid, the Yang may have a problem anchoring into the Yin and it begins floating to the surface of the body, triggering a hot flash or heavy sweat in the middle of the night. Using very hot herbs to strengthen the Yang solves the problem.

Fertility drugs, which also disturb the Yang rooting process in an abrupt manner, can have the same effect, forcing the Yang to the surface, and prompting hot flashes, or flickering of the Yang.

Because hot flashes can be symptomatic of another condition, Chinese medicine always recognizes that each patient must be treated individually. In fact, hot flashes and sweats can be caused by the opposite of Yang deficiency: by excessive heat accumulating in the Yang Ming sphere that drives Yang energy and body fluids outwards toward the exterior. Very cold formulas, like white tiger decoction with ginseng, are used to treat this condition.

A patient who was a medical doctor had been using hormone replacement therapy for several years to control her hot flashes. She sought my assistance in helping her discontinue the hormone treatments, but when she stopped, the hot flashes came on at a relentless pace. She could barely function as a physician. Normally, I would consider a case like hers a Yang deficiency, but after considering all the symptoms she displayed, it became clear that even though she was forty-six years old, it was a case of too much heat building in the Yang Ming. I gave her the white tiger decoction with ginseng, and two weeks later the symptoms were completely gone. The patient did not use hormone replacement therapy again.

The strength of Chinese medicine is the individual assessment of each patient. In today's world of Western medicine, all women who suffer from hot flashes are treated with the same hormones. Even in modern Chinese medicine, the situation is the same. Hot flashes and night sweats are considered to be the same Yin deficiency for all patients and are treated with the same herbs. *The Yellow Emperor* says that observing a symptom and automatically attaching to it a formula is the lowest form of medicine. In most cases, this treatment will prove itself wrong. Each patient has to be individually examined and the symptoms analyzed.

The same is, of course, true when it comes to solving infertility. Each person is unique and different. That is why we have our own different genetic codes, fingerprints, emotions, and desires. We need to see the difference in us to realize that there is no one drug that is good for everyone, and no one herb that is good for any one symptom.

ACUPUNCTURE – 365 POINTS WHERE ENERGY GATHERS

The doctor who sat facing my desk said, "Correct me if I am wrong. As far as I know, acupuncture is the use of needles to stimulate a network of energy channels. When you stick needles in certain points, it triggers the energy to circulate in the energy channels and thus it helps the patient recover." I had only one minute to explain myself before the next patient would step into the room. I had no choice but to reply that this was partially true. In fact, the doctor's understanding of acupuncture was not very complete at all. He had a very basic understanding of acupuncture but did not know the inner workings and complexities of the treatment.

The main classical work in Chinese medicine that pertains to acupuncture is the *Ling Shu*, also known as *The Yellow Emperor's Miraculous Pivot—Nine Needles and Twelve Origins*, where it is written "The crossing of joints have 365 gatherings. The meaning of 'joints' is the traveling, exiting and entering of the spirit and Qi. It is not the skin, flesh, tendons and bones."

This quote describes the points where true energy and the spirit gather. The true energy comes from the food we eat, while the spirit comes from the interaction between heaven and earth within our body. This gives us the first glimpse into what acupuncture is all about. When we insert needles into one of these points, we influence our own energy and influence the connection of our body with heaven and earth, or with our spirit.

While the body's true energy is inside our body, the 365 acupuncture points are the doors where the external heaven and earth energies—the three Yin and the three Yang—are waiting to enter. They are led inside by the spirit, known as Shen Ji. When the inside energy is strong and healthy, it will harmonize with the external energy. But when the internal energy is weak or ill, then there will be disharmony between the energies and we become ill.

There are many aspects I consider when determining in which acupuncture point to place a needle. A modern-day analogy is going to the airport to catch a flight. I plan my transportation to the airport. If I decide to take my car, I must know where to park and how to proceed to the terminal from the parking lot. I should know what I will need at the security checkpoint, which gate my flight is leaving from, how many bags I am allowed, and so much more.

In the practice of acupuncture, I need to be aware of the energies outside the body at the time of treatment. Is it a full moon or empty moon? Is it spring or fall? What are the dominant and guest energies at present? I must know the situation inside the patient. Is the liver energy strong or weak? Is the fire too strong or the water too weak? Then I must decide which acupuncture points I should use, how deep the needles should be placed, how much the needles should be rotated, and in which direction they should point.

Miraculous Pivot states: "You can't head on the coming and you can't pursue the going." This means that when the entering energy is too strong, the practitioner cannot increase available energy with acupuncture, and when the heaven's energy is departing, the practitioner can't sedate with acupuncture, because the inside energy is growing weaker. The state of one's health is always the result of an interaction between the inside energy and the outside world. This is fundamentally different than Western medicine. This is why there is a difference between Western drugs and herbs, and between surgery and acupuncture. Western medicine deals with the body as an independent unit, while Chinese medicine does not separate the body from nature.

The behavior of energy is universal. The heaven's three Yin and three Yang outside our bodies contain the same components as does the energy inside our body. In modern Chinese medicine, it is falsely perceived that the six heavenly influences—wind, cold, damp, dryness, warmth, and summer heat—are the cause of symptoms in our body.

It is actually the three Yin and three Yang inside our body that create the symptoms. This means that when cold enters, we can have cold symptoms, such as aversion to cold, or we can have hot symptoms, such as fever, or we can have dry symptoms like dry mouth and lips. This is because energy enters the body and then transforms within our own three Yin and Yang.

Why is there a therapeutic effect when inserting a needle into the body? This question is very illusive and its answer is very difficult to comprehend. In modern acupuncture, considerable scientific research has been done into the efficacy of acupuncture. However, the common approach is from the perspective that acupuncture works by stimulating the nervous system—efficacy must work on the physical level of nerves, flesh, skin, and bones.

An infertility patient sits in my office and tells me the following: In addition to irregular periods, she has a problem with depression in the spring. In the summer, she tends to gain weight, while in the winter she loses weight. All of these symptoms are contrary to what most other people generally experience. Now, which acupuncture points should we use and in what way?

We must consider that the spring is when the Yang energy rises. It is the wood energy of the Jue Yin and the warmth energy of Shao Yang. Depression is the emotion of fall, of metal and the lungs. The metal's job is to control the wood. Overactive wood will demand much of the metal. Because the outside energy of the spring enters our body via spirit and 365 gatherings, the wood becomes strong and the metal weak. Given that the patient feels depressed in spring, the outside energy is clearly impacting the inner three Yin and Yang. The summer belongs to fire and fire controls metal. The weak metal is overcontrolled in the summer and is weakened even more. The lungs are Tai Yin and together with the spleen, they are responsible for food metabolism. In the summer, the patient gains weight because the Tai Yin is impaired. In the fall and winter, the energy descends and helps the metal downward movement, thus making the metal and Tai Yin stronger, and the metabolism improves.

From this analysis, we can learn what needs to be strengthened and what needs to be reduced. The lung's metal is weak and liver wood is too strong, overcontrolling the spleen earth further, weakening the metabolism in the summer. However, in addition to strengthening the lungs and spleen and reducing the liver, we must consider the seasons. In the fall, we must strengthen the lungs metal and in the spring we must reduce the liver wood. In the summer, we must moderate the heart fire. We must consider the inside and outside of the problem.

UNDERSTANDING ACUPUNCTURE AND HOW IT RELATES TO DISEASE

Miraculous Pivot says: "Yin and Yang have different names, however, they are of the same kind. Above and below gather to penetrate through the meridians and side channels in an endless cycle. When evil energy attacks the patient, it can enter into the Yin or enter into the Yang. Above and below, right and left, they all have different reasons for attacking. When deficient evil enters the body, it alters the physical shape; however, when upright evil enters the body, one can only see slight changes in color.

The changes cannot be seen in the physical body, as if it is sometimes there and sometimes not, as if there are sometimes physical changes and at other times not."

This quote explains the relationship of our energy to heaven's energy and how disease comes about. Yin and Yang mean the energy inside and outside the body. The energies of heaven are above, and the inside energies are below. Our energy and heaven's energy combine to create the energy in the channels. This is why the spring can influence us in one way, while the summer will influence us in a different way. The summer will cause one patient to gain weight and the winter will cause the same patient to lose weight. Above and below, or inside and outside, energies will gather to penetrate through the meridians and side channels.

A modern approach to acupuncture is that each point has a specific action—one point is good for the tendons while another is effective for the uterus. This is not acupuncture the way the sages intended. When I hear a statement such as "This acupuncture point helps increase the blood flow to the uterus," I can only raise an eyebrow in dismay.

I believe that Chinese medicine must be integrated with Western medicine, because both have strong points, but I don't believe that Chinese medicine should be compromised in order to do so. In my practice, I collaborate with Western doctors on a regular basis. They work with me because they see results. The same goes for me. When I see results, I am likely to agree to work with the doctor involved. However, results for me do not mean that patients are conceiving, but rather that they are conceiving as naturally as possible.

Some of the 365 acupuncture points are more potent than others, at least from the angle of harmonizing heaven and earth with man. These are the Shu (transport) points.

Shu also means to bring a tribute from one place to the other. The character Shu is composed of two components. One is a cart with wheels and the other is a boat, meant to signify that a tribute can be brought via land or sea. *Miraculous Pivot – Nine Needles and Twelve Origins* states: *"The Yellow Emperor* asked: 'I heard that the five Yin organs and the six Yang organs have a place where they exit?' Qibo answered: 'The five Yin organs have five Shu each, and the six Yang organs have six Shu each. Five times five is twenty-five and six times six is thirty-six. Where the Shu exits, it is called Jing, where it trickles away it is called Ying, where it pours, it is called Shu, where it is marching, it is called Jing and where it enters, it is called He. The energy interaction of heaven and earth in the twenty channels and side channels are all in these five Shu points.'"

The main acupuncture points that harmonize the entering of

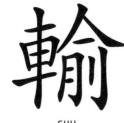

SHU

heaven energy and the exiting of body energy, then, are below the elbows and knees.

In traditional acupuncture, each acupuncture point has a Chinese name. In the West we have erased all the names because it was too difficult to remember for non-Chinese speakers, names such as Da Dun, Xing Jian, and Tai Chong now referred to as "liver 1, liver 2, liver 3." Each of the five Yin organs—lungs, heart, liver, spleen, and kidneys—has a meridian, and each of these meridians have five different types of Shu points: Jing, Ying, Shu, Jing and He. The third point on each meridian is the main Shu point, which carries the name of the entire group of points.

Exiting and trickling from the fingers and toes upwards, and entering and marching from the elbows and knees downwards, the heaven energy and the body energy pour and merge together at the Shu point. Among the five Shu points along the meridian, the Shu point is the third point or the middle point. It is the third point from the elbow down or the third point from the fingertip up. It is the center of the action. Heaven and earth are mixing together to enter the body at the Shu point and thus it is called Shu; to bring the tribute inside the body.

The characters Da and Tai are very similar and often interchange-

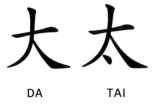

DA   TAI

able in classical Chinese. They both translate to big, huge, or extreme, and in ancient script they represent a human being. The character Da on the left is composed of two components. The horizontal line represents heaven and the two other lines represent man. The heaven crossing over the man means that the heaven and man are merging together. In the character Tai, there is also a small extension at the bottom of the foot signifying roots going into the ground.

When we look at the names of the five Yin organs Shu points (third point on each Yin meridian) and their corresponding organs, we can understand the difference.

Tai Yuan – lungs
Da Ling – heart
Tai Chong – liver
Tai Bai – spleen
Tai Xi – kidneys

We can see that each Shu point on each Yin meridian has the meaning "big"; however, the heart has "Da" and the other four organs have "Tai." We know that out of the five elements—wood, fire, earth, metal and water—only the fire is formless and flares upwards. All the other elements have physical forms and substance, and therefore, will gravitate downward toward the earth. The sages want to show us that within the five Shu points of the organs, the heart is purely connected to heaven with "Da," while the other four Shu points are connected to heaven too, but already gravitate to the earth with "Tai."

Now why would the Shu points of the Yin organs be "big"? This is, as we explained before, the place where the heaven's energy merges with the body's energy, hence it is a big place.

When we talk about the five Shu points, we must also know that the sages attributed the five elements to these points. For the Yin meridians, the distribution is as follows:

Jing – wood
Ying – fire
Shu – earth
Jing – metal
He – water

The Shu points are earth element. The sages realized that the heaven energy mixes with man's energy on the Yin meridians on the earth points. This distribution is not random. It is rather a description of natural phenomena. Our human energy comes from the Yin organs, and when it surfaces to the meridian, it exits at the Jing, trickles at the Ying, and becomes the biggest at the Shu earth point on that same meridian. From the other side, the heaven's energy enters at the He point, increases, or marches, at the Jing (this Jing is a different character than the first Jing even though it is pronounced the same) and becomes the biggest at the Shu earth points where it merges with human energy.

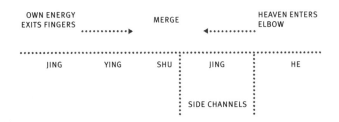

In the meridian system, Luo, or side channels, is where the meridians connect with each other. It is also where the energy splits off, entering our body from the meridians. When we look at the Yin meridians we discussed above, we can see that the side channel always starts either between the Shu-Jing points or between the Jing-He points.

The location where the energies mix is full or abundant, allowing the energy to enter into the body's deeper layers.

When standing upright with arms dropped, the elbows, where heaven's energy enters, are high, and the fingers, where human energy exits, are low. Similarly, the knees are high and the toes are low. High reaches to heaven and low reaches to the earth.

When the mixed energy enters the body, it is distributed within the body's three Yin and Yang, mixing with food energy and breathing air energy to become blood and nutrients to sustain our health. *Miraculous Pivot—Pathogenic Qi Zang Fu Organs, Disease and Physical Form* says, "All types of small pulse show that the Yin and Yang, physical form and Qi are deficient. You can't use acupuncture to treat it, but rather you have to use sweet herbs to strengthen it." According to *Miraculous Pivot – Beginning and End*, "If the Qi is not enough, the different pulses on the neck and wrist are all small. This is because the Yin and the Yang are both deficient. If you tonify the Yang with acupuncture, the Yin dries up, and if you drain the Yin, the Yang will separate. At this time you can use sweet herbs."

"Sweet herbs" does not necessarily mean herbs that are sweet. Sweet is the flavor of earth, the place where the myriad things are born. Sweet herbs means herbal formulas in general and herbs from the earth instead of acupuncture. When the Yin and Yang are deficient and when the Qi and blood are not enough, herbs must be used because they store the heaven's five essences and bring them into the five Yin organs. Acupuncture, on the other hand, harmonizes the heaven energy with the body energy, treating deficient and upright evil. Clearly both acupuncture and herbs are very useful in assisting infertility.

164

When needling a patient, the practitioner's intentions must be fully present or else the treatment is useless. *Miraculous Pivot—Beginning and End* states, "The intentions of your spirit lead will into the needle. For male on the inside and for female on the outside. Strengthening to prevent exiting and protecting to prevent entering. This is called reaching the Qi (De Qi)." For treatment to be effective, the practitioner must reach the Qi, which in Chinese is De Qi, by using his heart intentions and spirit to guide his will into the needle. For a male patient, the practitioner intentions must go inward, because male is Yang and his energy naturally wants to travel outwards. For a female patient, the practitioner intentions must travel outside, because female is Yin and her energy naturally wants to travel inward. The practitioner intentions aim to strengthen the upright energy of the patient, preventing it from exiting, and enabling it to prevent the evil energy from entering.

The correct movement of energy, entering or exiting, can be controlled. When I administer acupuncture, the patient can feel gurgling in the stomach, electricity running along the channel, heaviness, tingling, and pressure. Also, the area around the needle becomes 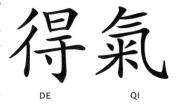 red. This is all part of the concept of De Qi. However, if the patient is very deficient in Yin and Yang, she will not feel any sensation and acupuncture is not beneficial. Rather, she needs herbal formulas to strengthen the Yin and Yang first, and then recommence acupuncture. Herbal formulas should be composed of raw herbs and not capsules or other patent pills that are depleted of heaven's energy.

For the Qi to arrive and for the acupuncture to be effective, the acupuncture needle must be inserted in the correct location. *Miraculous Pivot—Pathogenic Qi Zang Fu Organs, Disease and Physical Form* says, "*The Yellow Emperor* asked: 'what is the correct method of acupuncture?' Qibo answered: 'The needle must be placed in the Qi hole. It must not be placed in the muscles and joints. Needling the Qi hole will cause the needle to float in its harbor. Needling the muscles and joints will cause the skin to ache and the disease will aggravate.'"

As we explained before, the 365 acupuncture points are the junctions where the heaven's energy mixes with the body's energy. For the energy of the body to emerge, or for the energy of heaven to enter, one must needle these 365 points exactly. The points, what the emperor calls "holes," can be felt by palpating with the finger, and are between the muscles and joints, or between different muscles and tendons, so that the energy can gather. When we needle these holes, the energy can go one way or another, scattering or gathering, exiting or entering. Some of these "holes" are very small and hard to detect, some are large and easy to feel, but the experienced acupuncturist can feel them all.

The He points at the elbows and knees are big and deep, distributed on a large area of the skin. They contain the vast Yang energy, which, while entering, will become increasingly more condensed. The Jing points at the finger/toe tips are small and superficial, and they contain the condensed Yin energy which will gradually expand. They march toward each other, meeting at the middle Shu point. Yin and Yang are opposite in character and this is the natural way of heaven.

The needling depth is very important too. *Miraculous Pivot*: "When the Qi is in the meridian, the evil Qi is on top, the turbid Qi is in the middle and the clear mist Qi is at the bottom. When the needle is placed superficially, the evil comes out, when the needle enters midway, the turbid matter comes out, when the needle is too deep, the evil Qi to the contrary enters inwards and the disease aggravates."

This quote is telling us that the depth of the needle's puncturing is important and will affect the success or failure of the process. If the needling is too shallow, the body's energy will not exit. Turbid energy refers to the individual's own Yin energy, while evil Qi refers to heaven's Qi, as in deficient evil or upright evil. If one enters with the needle too deep, not only will the energy fail to emerge to mix with heaven's energy or to repel evil Qi, but it will cause the evil to enter.

When I hear about acupuncture courses of short duration such as medical acupuncture, which is a course for physicians ranging between 150–300 hours, I feel that a great disservice is being done to patients. I am also chagrined by the claims that medical acupuncture is superior to acupuncture administered by acupuncturists who have thousands of hours of training. On the other hand, I am also aware of medical doctors who receive real acupuncture training for three years, which makes them competent acupuncturists as well as medical doctors. This, I believe, is honorable and the patient should note the difference between the two.

ACUPUNCTURE: CHANNELING NATURE'S ENERGY INTO THE FERTILITY ZONE

Miraculous Pivot says: "The twelve meridians are where a person is born. It is where a disease culminates. It is where a person is healed. It is where disease arises. The acupuncture novice will begin his learning with this and the accomplished acupuncturist will end his study with it. A low-level practitioner finds it easy, while a master practitioner finds it very difficult. The first will frequent his mistake while the latter dwells on it as not to go wrong."

The twelve meridians are where heaven's energy enters and the body's energy exits. It is where the two energies merge to form and shape your health and longevity. When you have energy, you are born. Without energy, you have no life. This is true for the mother and father as well as for the new baby. Furthermore, the intricacy of the *Miraculous Pivot* text reveals a much deeper idea than the sages conveyed to us. The author conceals a special message in the first four sentences: A person is born, disease culminates, a person is healed, disease arises.

"Where a person is born" refers to our own energy. If our energy, three Yin and three Yang, is not healthy and harmonized, then a disease is already culminating. "Where a person is healed" refers to the external influence that enters and impacts our body. Disease will form and aggravate if we fail to control the exterior energy entering. The classics explain that the harmonizing of the internal energy or the control of the external energy all happens within the realm of the meridians. The meridians transform the three Yin and Yang. Therefore, an acupuncturist must always focus on learning as much as possible about these meridians.

The practice of acupuncture involves the spirit of the practitioner concentrating on the needle. The spirit, as we learned many times so far, is the vehicle for the entering and exiting of energy between heaven and man. When the practitioner connects the heaven's energy and his energy to the needle, we call this Qi arrival. Many of my patients comment that when they received acupuncture elsewhere they felt nothing, but in my acupuncture sessions they feel many strange sensations. They literally feel the energy moving at all times. My needles are not connected to any electrical outlets, only to my intentions. When I twist the needles I do not twist a piece of metal, but rather turn left and right, spring and fall, entering and exiting.

Miraculous Pivot explains, "The heaven is so high that you can't measure it and the earth is so wide that you can't weigh it. The person's life is born in between the heaven and earth. He is born within the six unifications. The heaven's height and earth's width, which is the root of his life, is not something that can be measured or weighed by man."

Dr. Jiao Shunfa, a famous Chinese neurosurgeon, invented scalp acupuncture in 1970 as a way to help stroke patients. His methods became so famous that the World Health Organization and the United Nations recognized scalp acupuncture as a major invention and recommended its method for clinical applications. But the story of scalp acupuncture was not always so famous and widespread. In 1984, a conference of neurosurgery department heads from all over China took place in Shanxi Province. A patient paralyzed in her right hand showed up at the outpatient clinic of the hospital where the conference took place. Dr. Jiao invited the neurosurgery chiefs to check the patient and come up with a diagnosis. The majority of doctors concluded that the reason for the paralysis was cerebral thrombosis, or blood clotting in the brain. When Dr. Jiao suggested to this group of senior doctors that scalp acupuncture would enable this patient to regain the ability to use her hand within five days, the crowd looked at him in disbelief. Dr. Jiao went further to predict that on the sixth day the patient would be able to roll dumplings with her hand. "If the patient does not recover her ability to use the hand as a normal person, I will stop practicing acupuncture," he told the dumbstruck audience. Five days later, the patient recovered full functionality in her right hand. On the sixth day, when Dr. Jiao arrived at the class, all the guest patients and doctors were gone. They had taken the patient to the cafeteria to check her ability to roll dumplings. When they came back to the conference hall, they all praised him for his success. From that day on, scalp acupuncture spread far and wide in China and around the world.

The practice of acupuncture for infertility is exactly like that. You can only believe it if you have seen it with your own eyes. Every day I see how patients improve and recover and become pregnant.

The acupuncture points that I use are below the elbows and below the knees. They are between point Jing at the finger/toe tips and He at the elbows and knees. The forearms and the lower legs are the location for the heaven's energy to enter, the body's Yin energy to exit, and the Yin and Yang to mix. *The Miraculous Pivot* says that heaven is Yang and the earth is Yin, and therefore the body's upper half corresponds to heaven and the body's lower part corresponds to earth. Thus the upper limbs correspond to heaven and the lower limbs correspond to earth.

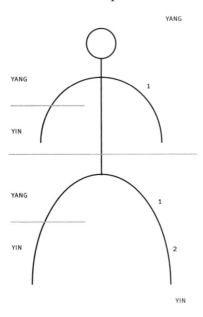

The lower legs are the Yin among the four limbs, while the forearms are the Yang. This is because the arms are close to heaven and correspond to Yang, and the legs are close to earth and correspond to Yin. Within the lower legs, the knees are the Yang within Yin and the toe tips are the Yin of Yin. As for the forearms, the fingers are Yin and the elbows are Yang. As explained earlier, the numbers occupy a special meaning. "Heaven 1 descends to create water, earth 2 ascends to embrace the fire, heaven 3 creates wood, and earth 4 creates metal." Numbers 1 and 2 represent the connection of heaven and earth and the connection to the pre-heaven state. Numbers 3 and 4 complement the first two in creating the post-heaven. In order to create harmony between our energy and heaven's energy, we need to use these four numbers. First, I must establish a connection between heaven and earth or between the outside energy and my body's energy. I use one needle at or around the elbow, which is the Yang of Yang. This brings the heaven's energy down into the body to create water. The water trigram has one solid Yang line in the center. One needle at the elbow represents this one Yang that creates the water. To bring the Yin energy of our body to exit and to mix with the Yang of heaven, I use two needles. I insert them close to the ankles, or at the Yin of Yin. I use the most Yin energy and two needles to create the effect of earth 2. This gives birth to fire. In the Li (fire) trigram we see that in order for it to take place, there are two solid Yang lines, one on top and one at the bottom. There is also one broken Yin line in the center. Two needles close to the ankles represent the broken line in the middle of the trigram. This is why the Classics say that Earth 2 gives birth to fire.

When I use two needles at the Yin of Yin, the body's own Yin energy exits to the surface to meet the heaven's energy. Under normal circumstances, this is what I want to reach with acupuncture. Heaven 1 is close to the elbow at the Yang of Yang, and earth 2 is close to the ankles at the Yin of Yin. The acupuncture points that I normally use are Tai Xi (vast brook/kidney 3) and San Yin Jiao (crossing of three Yin/spleen 6) if the patient is at her first fourteen days of the menstrual cycle. If the patient is at the second half of the menstrual cycle, I substitute San Yin Jiao (spleen 6) with Fu Liu (repeated current/kidney 7). I avoid the use of San Yin Jiao (spleen 6) if there is a possibility that the patient is pregnant because it can induce a miscarriage.

The first two rules of Hunyuan acupuncture are heaven 1 and earth 2 mixing and creating fire and water. This is the pre-heaven state before life turns into the post-heaven state. Two needles at the ankles and one at the elbows already gives birth to three needles. It is enough to create a trigram, or a state of energy, which needs at least three lines as we have seen in the Li (fire) and Kan (water) trigrams. The father of Daoism, Lao Zi, wrote in his book *Dao De Jing*: "One gives birth to two, two give birth to three, and three give birth to the myriad things." We need one of heaven and we need two of earth and together they are three. Water and fire together establish the pre-heaven connection. But we need the post-heaven state. We need the physical world we live in. We need the wood and the metal. We need the 3 and the 4.

To create this effect with acupuncture, I need a third needle on the leg in addition to the heaven 1 and earth 2. Heaven 1 and earth 2 comprise the vertical line of Jing, but I need the Wei horizontal line as well. This time I use the Yang of Yin or points close to the knee. As explained, 1 and 2 are descending and ascending to create water and fire (Sheng Jiang), while 3 and 4 are right and left and are also exiting and entering (Chu Ru). Three is the number giving birth to the east while 4 is the number giving birth to the west. In the east, the sun rises and we call this "sun exits from the earth." In the west the sun sets down. We call this "sun enters into the earth." This is what 3 and 4 exiting and entering means. The sun rises in the morning and the spring comes out after the winter. These two phenomena are the beginning of life. This is why the number 3 is the beginning of the post-heaven state; the state of life as we know it. The third needle of the leg gives new meaning to the harmony for which we strive. The 1 needle and the 2 needles mix the water and fire to create life's energy. However, we need the sunrise of spring needle. This third needle of the leg causes the mixed energy to spread in the body.

After we establish the use of three needles to bring the mixed Yin-Yang energy to spring into the body, we must plan our exit. We cannot have the sun rising without setting down, nor can we have the spring arriving without the fall to follow. This is a universal rule of our post-heaven state. Without left and right, and without entering and exiting, we find ourselves in the pre-heaven state—before life.

For the "exit" to come about, we do need four needles, but the fourth needle in acupuncture was already established when we entered the third needle of the leg—it is the needle in the arm that makes four needles. When I enter into the realm of the third needle, entering into the post-heaven state, there is already an "end" in sight. The pre-heaven state of heaven and earth is eternal. There is no end to it. But our life of post-heaven and right and left, east and west, entering and exiting is a state with an "end." When I insert the spring with the third needle, I have already established a post-heaven state with an "end" or "exit."

This means that with the third needle, I must be able to look far into the future. I am not inserting the needle to solve an immediate symptom, but creating the beginning of a long life cycle to come.

The one needle of the arm and three needles of the leg work in different ways on different areas, but I must have oversight of the entire action. The harmony of the four needles is crucial. This is dissimilar with Western medicine where a specialist will treat one problem and only one problem. With four needles, I need to solve the problems at hand and make sure that other problems will not arise in the future as a result of the acupuncture I perform. Sometimes I see acupuncturists inserting ten or twenty needles in all parts of the body without any logic or rules. The classics say that inserting needles at random without knowledge or correct purpose can inflict great harm.

ACUPUNCTURE AND PREGNANCY

Lao Zi, in his book *Dao De Jing* says: "Dao gives birth to 1, 1 gives birth to 2, 2 gives birth to 3 and 3 gives birth to the myriad things." Myriad things means everything under heaven: mountains, rivers, animals, plants, men, women, and babies. "3" gives birth to all of these. So what are these 1, 2, and 3?

Dao is the core principle for life and is the invisible part we need our heart to envision. This invisible Dao principle gives birth to the sun. Out of the sun comes the Yang energy needed for all life forms to exist. Second to that, and in extreme opposite side to it, we have the earth star, making only two orbits within a sixty-year period. Because this star is the farthest away from Yang and the sun, it has the least Yang energy. At the same time, it has the minimum Yang energy required for movement. The minimum movement of the earth star and the maximum Yang energy of the sun is the relationship needed to begin life. Thus Lao Zi said 1 gives birth to 2.

This relates directly to the human ability to become pregnant and begin a new life cycle. "1" gives birth to 2 means the male

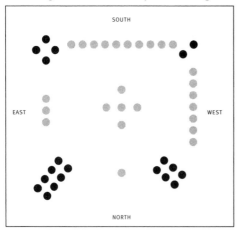

energy goes into the female body. 1 and 2 are on both extremes. But this by itself is not enough to create "everything under heaven." That is why Lao Zi said that 2 must give birth to 3 and then 3 can give birth to the myriad things.

The wood and fire stars are to the left of earth, and metal and water stars are to the right. This gives our planet and our life the balance we call Yin and Yang. It is not that the stars give us this balance, but rather that these stars follow the principle that we are to follow as well. The sages did not believe that the stars were influencing us, but rather the stars serve as the database, giving us the information we need to be able to use our heart to see the invisible principle of Yin and Yang. Even though our earth is in the middle between wood, fire, metal, and water, we are even more in the middle between the sun and the earth star. There are three celestial bodies to our right and three to our left. These are what the Yellow Emperor called the three Yin and three Yang.

When we start talking about "3," there is a more complex relationship. It is no longer just Yin and Yang, but rather Yin and Yang plus one other thing.

This new relationship is between the two extremes and the axis. The two extremes are the sun and the earth star, and the axis is our planet earth. We can clearly see that wood, fire, metal, and water distribute on both sides of the axis. The spring and summer are to our left and the fall and winter to our right. When we begin having this kind of a relationship, we call it "life." We have the most Yang source on the one hand and the most Yin source on the other, and in the middle we must have the axis for both of them. When these three come together we can say that the myriad things are born.

In the book of changes, *Yi Jing*, it is said that when the male and female essences exchange, the myriad things are born. The father is on the right and the mother on the left. The two come together to exchange their essence in order to create the center axis, a new wheel of Yin and Yang forming. This is called an embryo. This embryo axis starts revolving in an opposite direction, counter-clockwise, until becoming a baby, emerging out of the mother ten months later.

This 1, 2, and 3—or father, mother, and an axis—is the fundamental basis for conception. For this, we need the Yang energy to be in storage and to grow stronger. After pregnancy has been established, we must learn how to maintain and to nurture it so a healthy baby will be born.

In the Chinese language, the word *Zhi*, or cure, literally means "to control." When the above 1, 2, and 3 travel in a wrong direction, the doctor's job is to put it back on track. In today's "pregnancy world," Western doctors feel obligated to constantly

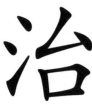

ZHI

intervene with blood tests and examinations. Many drugs and supplements are given to the pregnant woman. In Chinese medicine, the more a woman progresses with her pregnancy, the less treatment she needs.

However, a woman may need help conceiving because her conditions are not optimal. A pregnancy, aside from having a connection to the five elements and the numbers as we previously discussed, must be connected to the moon's principle, and if it isn't, there can be problems.

Miraculous Pivot–Discussion of Revealing the Year says, "A man is a reflection of heaven and earth. He reacts to the sun and the moon. Therefore, when the moon is full, the ocean is full to the west, the person's energy and blood are accumulating, and his hair, skin, and flesh are all supple. At this time, evil can attack only on a superficial level. When the moon is empty, the ocean is full to the east, the person's energy and blood are depleted, his defenses are down and his body stands alone in the fight. His hair, skin, and flesh are deficient. At this time, evil can attack to a deeper level."

We can see that the sages understood the relationship between the moon and our body. The opening statement says that the human body reacts to the sun and the moon movements.

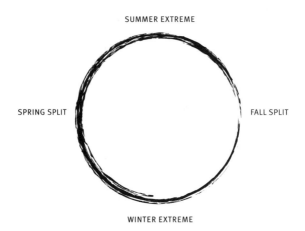

SUMMER EXTREME

SPRING SPLIT

FALL SPLIT

WINTER EXTREME

In the Chinese lunar calendar, the year is divided into twenty-four segments. Each segment is approximately two weeks long. Even though it is a lunar calendar, it is divided according to the sun's movements. The sun travels every year from north to south, back and forth. When the sun arrives at the most southern point, it is referred to on the calendar as Dong Zhi or "winter extreme." When the sun returns toward the north and crosses the equator, it is called Chun Fen, or "spring split." When the sun continues its travel to the north until its most extreme point, it is referred to as Xia Zhi, or "summer extreme." When the sun then travels back southward and crosses the equator again, it is referred to as the Qiu Fen, or "fall split." The sun's circular motion establishes the four seasons. The entire planet reacts to the sun accordingly.

The same is true with the moon, but on a different platform. The moon orbits our planet earth every 29.5 days and circles around itself every 29.5 days, creating a special phenomenon, enabling us to view the same side of the moon all the time.

When the moon is full, it contains all the Yang energy. This is similar to the storage of Yang in our body. We can also use this principle to learn about the development of our pregnancy and baby art is covering descender.

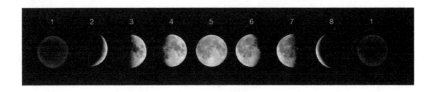

The moon has eight phases, but for simplification purposes, we will divide it into four phases to match the four seasons. An empty or new moon is 1, the half moon growing is 3, the full moon is 5, and a half moon waning is 7. Thereafter, it is back to an empty moon 1. The new moon always rises at sunrise. The first half moon rises at noon. The full moon rises at sunset. The waning half moon rises at midnight. From this, we can see that the moon behaves differently depending on the amount of Yang energy within it. When the moon begins filling up with Yang energy, it rises at sunrise and when it is full with Yang energy (full moon) it rises at sunset.

This is very significant. Let's imagine that the moon is an energy tank where the "Yang energy reserves" are kept. When this tank is empty, it fills up on the sun's energy when the sun is in the sky. By the time the sun disappears, the tank is full and the tank is able to provide energy for light.

The Yellow Emperor says that we react to the sun and the moon. We wake up every morning for sunrise using new Yang energy, and we charge our energy every night when we go to sleep. The moon relates to our ability to recharge, or bring the Yang energy into storage. When the moon is full, it rises at sundown and stays with us throughout the night. This is why the Yellow Emperor says that when the moon is full, the energy and blood are full and evil can enter only at a superficial level, but when the moon is empty, the energy and blood are weak and evil can enter deep into the body.

A woman's menses preferably occurs when the moon is empty and the energy and blood are weakest. Her ovulation should occur when the moon is full and her energy and blood are at peak strength. The time for successful conception is when the moon is full. However, women often get their periods at different times of the lunar cycle.

In the classics, the sages stated that when the woman's period is irregular, the practitioner must regulate it in order for the woman to be healthy. Modern practitioners believe that the sages meant to regulate menstruation by making it occur every twenty-eight days. The sages, however, meant that a regular menstruation is a period conforming to the moon cycle.

Synchronization with the moon happens on its own if all conditions are met. A person who follows nature is healthy and a healthy person is in sync with the moon naturally. However, one thing a person can do is follow the lunar cycles in his or her behavior, so when the moon is full, he or she should be more outgoing, and when the moon is empty, more reserved and withdrawn.

Synchronization with the lunar cycle is extremely important for pregnancy. The reason the body allows pregnancy is because our cycle is in sync with the moon and sun, with the ability to store Yang energy. When the body functions well, it knows that the baby can be healthy and it allows the woman to conceive. The system of male sperm and female ovum and the essence behind them is extremely potent. If the body is correctly storing Yang energy, the sperm and ovum have no problem finding each other. If Yang storage is impaired, then the code is broken and the essence is weak.

We must understand that if the body is not healthy, then it is not in a position to become pregnant or to keep a healthy pregnancy. When young children are sickly, it can partially be blamed on poor lifestyle and diet, but it is also because a pregnant mother couldn't harmonize with the lunar Yang storage phases.

The locations of moonrise and moonset at the horizon show the same variation during a month that the locations of sunrise and sunset do during a year. For those in the northern hemisphere, when the sun is in the south it is winter and when the sun is in the north it is summer. The same happens with the moon every month. The lunar rising and setting change locations, which impacts our ability to store Yang energy. One Qigong exercise, which is very effective, is to stand outdoors in the evening when the full moon comes out and simply watch the moon and inhale slowly, harmonizing with it. You can only do this exercise when the moon is full.

> While gazing at the full moon allow your mouth to fill with Jade water (saliva), then swallow the jade water in three portions, after each swallow imagine that the moon's light is entering your stomach. Exercise for 10–20 minutes.

The Yellow Emperor says that man (and woman) responds to the sun and the moon, and that the female reaction to the moon stops at around the age of forty-nine, meaning at menopause. The period can still come but the ability to conceive and create new life stops.

Aside from helping our body become strong every month by knowing the moon, we can also learn about the development of the baby during pregnancy. The female becoming pregnant is the result of the female acting as the Yin counterpart of the moon. Its action of regenerating storage is the story of the "new life." The way that it recharges reflects the way a baby is developing. When the moon starts as a crescent new moon, it appears at the northwest, or rather, the northwest part of the moon appears. This is the time when the baby is conceived. Thereafter, the moon gradually grows upwards toward the south and leftwards toward the east until the first growing half moon fills the right side of the moon (the west side). The moon continues to grow to become a full moon, which is the south, and this is midpregnancy. The moon then starts to wane down to the east (to the left).

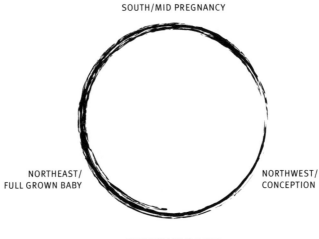

SOUTH/MID PREGNANCY

NORTHEAST/
FULL GROWN BABY

NORTHWEST/
CONCEPTION

NORTH/BABY IS BORN

The moon wanes until only the half moon remains at the east
(left side). Then the moon wanes to a declining crescent moon that
is visible at the northeast. At this time, the baby is fully grown and
ready to emerge. The last phase of the moon is an empty moon.
This is month ten of a pregnancy when the baby is delivered.

Premature babies are often healthy, but are generally slightly
less healthy than fully matured babies. This is because their five
directions are established in the first five months of pregnancy.

When we understand the two phases of a pregnancy, we begin
to have an insight into Chinese medicine miscarriage prevention
and how to treat a pregnant woman. A pregnancy has two phases
and not three trimesters as Western medicine pioneered. The first
phase is the first five months of pregnancy, which includes the pre-
conception phase. Infertility treatment falls under this category. I
treat the mother and the father not only so they can conceive, but
rather so that their creation will survive the first five months.

The doctor's job is to ensure that conception will get to a full
moon. He must have the vision that his treatment of infertility does
the job for at least the first half of the pregnancy. It is also his job to
make the second phase of the pregnancy proceed smoothly as well.

I had a patient who had suffered five miscarriages, three of which were during week fourteen, before coming to see me. In each case, she was treated with different Western medications unsuccessfully, but these medications could not correct her lunar cycle. Using herbs and acupuncture during the first phase of pregnancy, which restored harmony with the moon, she carried to term.

Before continuing with the two phases of pregnancy, I want to explain another point regarding fertility and successful conception, as this relates to phase one of pregnancy. The moon grows from the northwest to the south; however, our Yang energy opens up in the reverse direction, from northeast to the south. When the moon grows, the Yang energy increases because it increases the Yang energy storage. However, when the Yang energy opens up in the east or northeast, this starts the process of spending the Yang. At the same time, the spending of the Yang is a daily cycle, while the storage of the Yang as it relates to the moon is in monthly cycles.

When the storage of the moon is full, the body's overall energy and blood are full. This is the time for conception, or as Western medicine might put it, "ovulation." This time is in the south. At

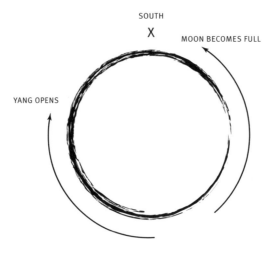

SOUTH

X

MOON BECOMES FULL

YANG OPENS

NORTH/NEW MOON/YANG RISE

the same time we must understand the other side of the chart. The north, or the time Zi, (11 P.M.–1 A.M.) is the Shao Yin time. It is the time of the emperor fire, when the heart's fire warms up the true Yang of the kidney's water. This causes the Yang energy to exit.

The east is the time of Mao (7 A.M. – 9 A.M.). It is the time of the Shao Yang's minister fire. The minister fire pushes the rising of the Yang energy until it gets to the south where it is most open and used up. In general, the Yang opening up combined with the full moon is the time where libido or sex drive peaks. It is the time of conception as well. This is why many women experience an increase in libido around the fertile time. "Sex drive" is connected to fertile time and reflects the health of the stored Yang. The seasons are spring and summer and correspond to the time when animals move into "heat" and are intent on reproducing.

After the male and female essences have exchanged and a new life is created, the whole process of the baby developing in the first five months is the process of the moon becoming full. The mother nurtures this process of establishing the child's five directions. In the second phase, when the directions are complete, the child begins to be demanding. In the baby's fetus world, the moon cycles are dominant, the rotation of the fetus moving counterclockwise from the northwest to the northeast.

Come month ten, the baby emerges into our world, his Yang revolution becoming the same as ours. It revolves clockwise from the northeast to the northwest. At this time, the baby's energy walks the same route as adults and the treatment must adapt accordingly.

In the first phase of pregnancy, the treatment goal is to help the baby as its five directions form. If anything is wrong with the harmony, we must help the child first. During the second phase, the moon declines. This means that the energy and blood of the mother decline. The job of the doctor in the pregnancy's second phase is to strengthen the mother and prepare her for delivery.

> I strengthen the mother with Chinese herbs and acupuncture, also by guiding her with diet and on how to stay away from harmful substances.

Of course, strengthening the baby is no less important, but one should remember that the five directions have been established and simply need to be completed, represented by the numbers 6, 7, 8, 9, and 10. In the first phase, the mother creates the baby's five directions, while in the second phase the baby pulls from the mother the resources needed for its completion. In this second phase, it is most common to see a pregnant woman diagnosed by Western doctors with gestational diabetes or anemia. In reality, this is a natural process and it merely means that the mother's resources are overtaxed by the baby.

The first phase and second phase of pregnancy is the designation made by the sage to ensure a healthy future generation. The first phase of pregnancy is called the pre-heaven phase, while the second is called the post-heaven phase. During the pre-heaven the mother is giving and during the post-heaven the mother is taxed by the baby.

The Yellow Emperor explains that the minister fire comes down to earth to create fire, shaping the 10,000 shapes and forms. The emperor fire, or "heaven's essence," doesn't come down to earth. Instead, it reaches the Yin organs and is stored as essence. When form (Xing) and essence (Jing) unite, we get "birth" (Sheng Hua). In this context "form" refers to the female ovum and the male sperm, and what we call "essence" refers to the mother's and father's Shao Yin. The man reflects the heaven and earth, and so he has the heaven's Yang essence as well as the earth's Yin form.

184

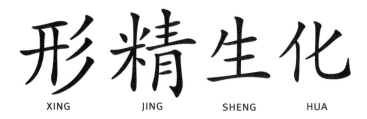

XING   JING   SHENG   HUA

There is the form and the essence. The form alone can't do the job, nor can the essence. The Yellow Emperor says that the kidneys rule the storage of essence. The kidneys in Chinese medicine are the Shao Yin emperor fire. The essence that the Yellow Emperor is talking about is the essence that can give birth to a new life. It is the essence of the five directions: north, south, east, west, and center, the same five directions needed to establish the first phase of pregnancy and the first five numbers of the baby—1, 2, 3, 4, and 5. This whole dynamic explains what the emperor means when he says that minister fire comes down to the earth and emperor fire does not. The minister fire is the fire creating the "form," or sperm and egg. The emperor fire is the fire stored as essence that we call Shao Yin essence. This is why we say that the man reflects the heaven and earth and he has two fires.

Minister fire leads the Yang and emperor fire pilots the Yin. Our Yin energy is the heaven's energy stored in our body as essence. The Yang energy is our body's functions. Therefore, when we treat a pregnant woman, we want to help the mother and the baby. To help the mother, we help the Yang energy and the minister fire, and to help the baby, we help the Yin or the emperor fire. Helping the Yin and baby is never ever clearing heat or using thick herbs to obstruct the Yang, the way it is widely practiced today. Yin is emperor fire. It is heaven Yang stored within the body as essence. Using acupuncture or herbs to obstruct the heaven's Yang and the Shao Yin is what the sages called "putting the patient under the sword of medicine."

ACUPUNCTURE PRINCIPLES AND GUIDELINES

During the first phase of pregnancy, the primary treatment principle is to help the baby; acupuncture is the preferred treatment modality. If the father and mother are not in optimal health at time of conception, then herbal formulas can be considered as well. What is most necessary, however, is neither acupuncture nor herbs, but rather Chinese medicine. Many think that herbs used in the Chinese herbal pharmacy equal Chinese medicine. This is not true. A cup of hot water could be Chinese medicine, while popular Chinese herbs like Dang Gui (Dang Quai) may not be. If the practitioner understands Yin and Yang well in the way that the sages did, he can use a cup of hot water to cure the patient. Speaking for myself, I have helped many of my pregnant patients recover with a cup of hot water.

Many patients in midpregnancy experience heartburn. Over-the-counter remedies are often prescribed by the obstetrician/gynocologist, but shouldn't be. When the baby grows in the uterus, the Ren and Chong meridians are obstructed and the stomach descending motion is hindered, heartburn as well as nausea and belching can result. Hot water is water with extra Yang energy. This is the Yang energy in water as described earlier in the book, represented by the water trigram.

When extra true Yang energy from hot water enters the stomach, the stomach can recover its natural function of descending and the heartburn stops.

The same is true with acupuncture. When the practitioner understands the nature of the problem, the number of needles used doesn't matter. If the acupuncturist does not understand the nature of the problem, then even twenty needles will not do the job.

The most important aspect, and at the same time the most difficult, is to know when it is best to treat a patient and when to avoid intervention. The basic and most fundamental principle of Chinese medicine is to restore balance. If the patient is already balanced, it is possible that treatment will put her out of balance. Some modern practitioners, when treating a patient, use Western methodologies to determine when to treat. They may decide to treat ovulation issues during the follicular phase and menstrual problems during the luteal phase. They may treat based on assessment of Yang energy according to basal body temperature. This kind of approach, however, is not Chinese medicine, but rather Western medicine with needles and herbs. With true Chinese medicine, the appropriate time for treatment is solely based on whether or not the patient is in harmony.

Along the same lines, the Western system often discovers pregnancy issues as a result of doing routine interventions or tests. Sometimes the mother and/or baby are already in trouble. In Chinese medicine, these issues are resolved before they happen, which is of course far preferable.

With regard to stopping and starting treatment when pregnant, if the patient feels uncomfortable symptoms, such as nausea, back pain, hemorrhoids, heartburn, or acid reflux, treatment can be very useful. Other symptoms, such as very mild nausea in the first phase, are normal and no treatment is needed.

ACUPUNCTURE, IVF, AND EVIDENCE-BASED SCIENCE

Acupuncture has made large strides in modern medicine. Today it is a popular treatment modality. Many health insurance companies now cover acupuncture treatments. Many medical doctors are referring their patients to acupuncture practitioners.

It is clear to me that the reason acupuncture has been found to be beneficial for IVF patients is that the acupuncture does make a woman healthier and more able to withstand the IVF procedure. However, these women who become healthier with acupuncture are just as likely to then go on and have a baby naturally as they are to start IVF procedures. Instead of supporting the IVF procedure, the acupuncture should be seen as a stand-alone answer. It is far less invasive, has far fewer side effects, and will not be as costly.

SUPERMARKETS OUT, LOCAL FARMS IN

The centralization of the food chain and the ruining of food with artificial ingredients can have a negative effect on our health and fertility, and its effects on future generations is as yet unknown. We have to make the right choices when it comes to our food.

The Chinese sage Sun Simiao named his classical book *Emergency Prescription Worth a Thousand Gold*, meaning the life and health of a person is most precious. But for whom is it precious? It is only precious for the individual himself. With regard to modern food, an individual's health is not precious to the big companies producing the food. Therefore, it is up to the individual to ensure quality. Of course, if manufactured food were to be harmful upon digestion, authorities would shut down the companies involved. But if food products are harmful over a period of many years, the companies are not held accountable and are safe to make their profits.

Big food companies have tremendous resources when it comes to manipulating public opinion. This can be done through advertising, government lobbying, and the sponsorship of "studies" that prove desired results.

How do we know what we should eat and where to get it? I think we should all look into our heart and find our belief. We should look for what makes sense to us that creates our belief. When my oldest daughter was born, I became very worried. I had an overwhelming desire to find out the truth about food and be able to give it to my family. I went on a difficult quest where I met controversy. It was difficult to know right from wrong, but I always fell back onto my heart. I looked for the warm place in there, where I asked myself, *what would my mother, grandmother, and great-grandmother have done? What would they decide?*

The answer has always been the same—to rely on the generations. They didn't choose what to buy at the market, or what to cook at home, because of a study they read. In today's world, we have stopped listening to our mother's voice. We are listening to science now.

We must go back to the time when the reason for cooking food was to make it delicious and healthy. It was a time when the mother would put love into cooking for her children and go out of her way to acquire the best possible ingredients. These are diets that have been created over many centuries for only one purpose: creating and sustaining a healthy next generation.

RECOMMENDATIONS OF THE GENERATIONS

We provide ourselves with an abundance of food year round. We can buy summer fruits in winter and tropical fruits in Alaska. Even though this may seem fine to the naked eye, it is not. When fruits and vegetable grow in a certain climate or in a certain season, they can supplement a real and current bodily need. If we eat a watermelon, which is watery and cool, in summer it can actually slow down the Yang expansion, restoring harmony in our body.

At this time, eating a watermelon is beneficial to our health. However, what happens when we eat a watermelon imported from South America in the middle of winter? Our Yang energy is in a contraction state in accordance with the winter season. A watermelon will overly shrink the Yang into contraction, harming the true Yang of the kidneys.

The Yellow Emperor says if it's hot, cool it off, and if it's cold, warm it up. This is how we strive back to harmony. This is why there are no cold fruits or vegetables growing in winter, when people should eat more animal food, such as meat and animal fat. This creates the energy needed to warm up the kidney Yang. There are many cold vegetables and fruits that grow in the summer, which can help cool us down when the heaven Yang descends with all its vigor and the dead winter earth is born into life. Because the live Yin energy of the earth is what fills up the plants and trees, the fruits and vegetable we eat contain an amount of Yin energy. This is why they are juicy. If one dries the fruits and vegetables, they become more Yang. Dry fruit, then, is not cold and can be eaten in the winter. The same is true with pickled fruits and vegetables.

> Eat fruits and vegetables in season, more in spring, summer and fall but less in winter. Eat meat and fat in winter and less in spring and summer. Eggs and dairy more in spring and fall but less in summer and winter. Eat and drink hot food in winter, spring and fall, but less in summer.

During the winter, Yang is sparse and the earth is dead. Animals have a longer life cycle than one year. They eat large volumes during the thriving spring and summer seasons, storing it in their body as fat reserves for the winter. The animal fat is condensed Yang that is then released gradually, warming and nourishing the animal throughout the winter, and is actually an expansion of the Yang mechanism.

Because meat and fat warm the Yang, we should eat less of it in the spring and summer and more of it in the fall and winter. This is the way to be harmonious with your diet. It has nothing to do with low fat and more veggies. The bottom line is that to eat certain food at the right time is good; to eat the same food at the wrong time is not. If you eat in accordance with the seasons, it will be beneficial for your health, but may not be beneficial for the food industry.

Our food must be regulated according to nature; to eat healthily, you must buy your food locally. The energy in the local farmer's produce is the best for your health, and is worth the extra few dollars you may pay.

Today's transportation and globalization give rise to many problems in our diet. There is wide consumption of a product referred to as soy protein, which acts as a substitute for meat. It is consumed by Westerners who should not eat it because it is often highly processed. Such a food can seriously offset Yin and Yang.

The second most important element in traditional diet is the food quality. It is not just that the additives and chemicals added to food are harmful, but the quality of the food itself is. If the food is of a good quality and unadulterated, the energy within is abundant. This will improve health and fertility substantially.

Many people lack the confidence in the food they are eating unless it is sold in a major chain food store. This is the wrong way to obtain food. You need to find out for yourself if what you eat is safe or not. You, not the store manager, must be in charge of your safety.

FRUITS AND VEGETABLES – BE SEASONALLY CORRECT

Fruits and vegetables are generally healthy if grown locally and in season. Consumption of fruits and vegetables in winter should be reduced and limited unless dried or pickled.

Vegetable oils are not the same as vegetables. Because they are unsaturated, if fried, they tend to oxidize and can be very harmful to your health and fertility. Unfortunately, many vegetable oils are already highly oxidized when purchased. For cooking, it is best to use saturated fat, such as chicken fat, lard, or butter. A few vegetable oils are good, but only if cold-pressed, organic, and used cold in salad dressing. It is important to read labels. Avoid food with vegetable oil listed as an ingredient. Processed fruits and vegetables with added chemicals, colors, and preservatives are not healthy.

EGGS AND POULTRY – FROM CHICKENS THAT EAT A NATURAL DIET

I believe we should strive to eat as naturally as possible to ensure optimal nutrients. Eggs that come from free-range chickens, for example, are more nutritional. Free-range means chickens that are free to roam, enabling them to eat worms and insects. Most organic growers feed organic grains to their chickens. Although this is preferable to genetically modified grains used by the mainstream poultry industry, it does not compare to free-range chickens. The result is seen in the eggs and yolks. The egg yolks from free-range chickens are dark yellow or dark orange.

Eating premium quality eggs supports nutrient intake. Premium quality egg yolks are particularly beneficial to your health.

Another good source of nutrients are chicken livers and bone marrow. The Chinese diet includes the entire chicken with the bones, skin and head, not just the meat. A chicken raised humanely in a healthy way is an excellent source of Yin and Yang energy.

MEAT AND FAT – SPARE THE GROWTH HORMONES

It is of great importance for consumers to know the source of the meat and animal fat they are consuming. Similar to chickens, healthy cows, sheep and goats will produce healthy meat and fat. The key to raising healthy animals is to maintain their natural habitat and diet. The fat and organ meat from grass-fed beef is much healthier than that of an animal that is fed grain, receiving growth hormones or antibiotics. Liver from grass-fed beef is especially recommended.

THE FOUR LEVELS OF THE HUNYUAN METHOD

While Chinese herbs and acupuncture are decisively not "do-it-yourself" modalities, I have long thought it would be beneficial to introduce a home program based on this ancient wisdom. With the Hunyuan method, I divide my treatment protocol into four levels. Approximately 25 percent of all pregnancies resulting from the Hunyuan Method are reached due to the first two levels of treatment. Approximately 75 percent of pregnancies result from all four levels. However, these include strong, potent herbs that are not recommended for home remedies as they can only be taken under strict supervision of a practitioner. Therefore, these potent herbs have been left out of the home program in favor of kitchen-based, mild herbs that carry no risk. The efficacy, of course, will not be the same as it would be if the patient visited an acupuncturist. However, to help improve the results of the mild herbs, I will explain additional methods of acupressure, Qigong exercises, and diet and lifestyle modifications. Again, this do-it-yourself protocol is not a substitute for visiting a health care professional or an herbalist, but it is your first step toward success.

It is recommended that each level be practiced for one month before proceeding to the next. However, if the patient does not suffer from any symptoms listed under Level One, she should proceed to Level Two immediately. If the patient is in the midst of levels two through four when a Yang illness or blockage arises, she must return to level one (or level two if level one is not applicable). When she has rebalanced the three Yang spheres at level one, within three days she may return to the level where the blockage began.

LEVEL ONE: BALANCING THE THREE YANG SPHERES: TAI YANG, SHAO YANG, YANG MING

Before Yang meets Yin—before the Tai Yang life force connects with the Yin energy force within the body—it is imperative that the three Yang life force energy spheres come into balance.

The balance for disharmony in the Tai Yang, Shao Yang and Yang Ming spheres must conform to the laws of nature: it must follow a natural modality of treatment such as offered by Chinese, Ayurvedic, or American Indian folk medicine. With Chinese medicine, the remedy for getting into balance consists of diet, herbs, acupressure, Qigong (therapeutic movement and/or breathing), emotional balancing, and lifestyle modifications.

TAI YANG ILLNESS

RECOGNIZING THE LIFE FORCE ENERGY IMBALANCE

Tai Yang illness occurs when the Yang mechanism—where the life force exits the body—is blocked from opening. The symptoms can be one or more of the following: chills, fever, runny or stuffed nose, stiff neck, general body aches and exhaustion.

Although these symptoms do not appear to constitute a serious Western medical illness, they are serious from a Chinese fertility perspective. If not treated, the disharmony can travel deep into the Shao Yin, possibly damaging fertility prospects.

BRINGING THE IMBALANCE BACK TO HARMONY

There are a number of steps necessary to remedy or balance the imbalance that is making you ill. These methods include a new diet, herbs, acupressure, Qi Gong, emotional adjustments, and a change in lifestyle. Modern cold remedies will force the illness to an inward place, causing it to become more serious.

194

DIET — LOSE THE DAIRY, EAT BLAND

Consumption of any dairy product, as well as oily, deep fried, spicy, and/or salty food, can obstruct the Tai Yang energy force. Cold food and beverages will dampen the heat of the Tai Yang fire.

Bland foods are recommended, such as sprouted bread, eggs, lightly cooked vegetables, and chicken soup. It is best to eat small quantities rather than large meals so as not to further exacerbate the obstruction.

HERBAL — SPREAD THE FIRE

Add three teaspoons cinnamon twigs (not cinnamon powder), three slices fresh ginger, and two teaspoons of maple syrup to two cups of water. Boil the mixture for twenty minutes.

In the early afternoon, drink one cup on an empty stomach, followed by a bowl of rice soup. Afterwards, lie down in a relaxed position under blankets. Help the life energy move through your body by imagining fire spreading from the heart to the extremities. Remain in this position until light perspiration forms on the skin.

ACUPRESSURE — STIMULATE ENERGY MOVEMENT

Use fingers to lightly stimulate the area around acupressure points GB 20 at the back of the neck, and Stomach 40 at the mid-shinbone on the lateral side (*see* appendix C on page 246 for illustrations of acupressure points mentioned in this chapter). It is not necessary to locate the exact points. Rub these areas three times per day.

QI GONG — RUB IT DOWN

When the Yang energy is blocked, it is advantageous to rub down the four extremities.

Stretch both hands in front of you, fingers pointing forward and away from the body. Insert the right thumb under the left armpit with four fingers hugging the top of the upper arm. Rub all the way down your arm and hand. Repeat the process twelve times. Switch to your right arm and do the same.

Use both hands to encircle your right upper thigh, close to the crotch, and rub down your leg and right foot. Repeat the process twelve times and then switch to your left leg.

EMOTIONAL — LEAVE THE STRESS BEHIND

Pensiveness means to think, think, think. This over-thinking restricts the Tai Yang from opening. Ease both the mind and body by retiring to bed and forgetting about everything. This will allow the life force to flow smoothly, uninterrupted.

LIFESTYLE — JUST HANG OUT

Do not exercise.

Do not work.

Avoid exposure to wind along the neck and its nape.

SHAO YANG ILLNESS

RECOGNIZING THE IMBALANCE

Shao Yang illness occurs when the Yang energy fails to warm up, and the Tai Yang is unable to ignite the fire.

The main symptoms of the Shao Yang illness are dry eyes, bitter taste in the mouth, slight nausea, a general feeling of discomfort in the chest and abdomen area, headaches on one side of the head or behind the eye, decreased appetite, an upset emotional state, and a wiry pulse.

ELIMINATING THE IMBALANCE

DIET — AVOID SUGAR STAGNATION

Stay away from sweets such as chocolate and jams. These foods create stagnation and drain the heat needed for the Shao Yang.

Include slightly cool spicy, salty, and sweet flavors, and moderate seasoning of all food.

Recommended: Beef soup with cilantro and mint.

Herbal – A trip to the garden

Add eight teaspoons rosemary, three pieces of fresh ginger, two tablespoons cut licorice root, and nine dandelion leaves to three cups of water. Boil the mixture for thirty minutes. Drink one cup at room temperature after morning breakfast.

Acupressure – Improve Yang energy circulation

External stimulation of the body can improve the circulation of the Yang energy. Relax both hands to the sides of the body. Clench fists lightly and place the eye of the fists (thumb and index finger) at GB 31 along the sides of thighs. Tap on GB 31 with your fists' eye twenty-four times. Repeat the process eight times per day.

Qi Gong – Radiate the life force

Use thumbs and eight fingers to brush through the hair from the forehead backwards toward the neck. Brush back on the sides of the head, returning to the forehead. Use slight force so as to feel the Yang energy traveling to your face. On waking in the morning, rub the scalp with medium force from front to rear twenty-four times, radiating the life force.

Emotional – Don't worry, be happy

Avoid anger and frustration. Add joy to your day, helping to kindle and sustain the Shao Yang fire.

Lifestyle – Stress-free mornings

The morning is when the Shao Yang is most active. Stressful mornings must be avoided in order to give the Shao Yang the balance it needs to do its work.

YANG MING ILLNESS

RECOGNIZING THE IMBALANCE

The body's life force needs rest. Yang Ming illness occurs when the Yang mechanism that facilitates the entrance of the life force back into storage cannot do so. The life force overstays its welcome.

When the life force cannot close down, symptoms include overheating, increased thirst and desire for cold drinks, constipation, constant hunger, red face, increased perspiration, strong and rapid pulse.

CORRECTING THE IMBALANCE

DIET — KEEP IT COOL

Avoid bread, rice, milk and other constipating foods, as well as greasy and/or deep fried foods.

Include: Raw and leafy vegetables such as spinach and cabbage.

If you are suffering from heat symptoms, or you are craving cold beverages, you may add cold drinks to your diet, but this should be discontinued once heat symptoms subside.

HERBAL — TASTES GREAT

Add two teaspoons of organic honey and ¼ teaspoon grated fresh ginger to one cup of hot water. Cool the beverage and drink late in the evening before going to sleep.

ACUPRESSURE

While in a sitting position, use the base of the palms to rub the point Stomach 32 forward and backwards thirty-six times. Apply four times a day.

QI GONG — UNLOCK THE GATES

This exercise helps to unlock the Yang Ming. The Yang is finally able to retreat into storage.

Layer palms on each other, placing them on top of abdomen. In a circular motion rub entire abdomen with medium pressure from the lower abdomen to the left side to the upper abdomen to the right side. Repeat for thirty-six rotations. Change direction for twenty-four rotations.

EMOTIONAL — GET THAT SMILE OFF YOUR FACE
Joy and laughter will increase the warmth around Tai Yang. It is best to keep the mind in an even mood of peacefulness.

LIFESTYLE — CUT DOWN ON EVENING STIMULATION
Excitement and stimulation during the evening hours will prevent the Yang Ming from closing down, the fire persisting. It is best to eat a light dinner and to go to bed early. Television and other stimulants should be avoided, although listening to soft music may calm your mind.

LEVEL TWO: STRENGTHENING THE TAI YIN SPHERE

As opposed to the Yang spheres, the Yin spheres are inside the body, from the cellular level to the organ level. The three aspects of the Yin—the Tai, the Shao and the Jue—compose the body's Yin energy. They contain the storage of old energy, the death of old energy, as well as transformation and rebirth of new energy.

The three Yin are the source of life and the root of fertility. The Tai Yin is the pure Yin, representing the earth as the mother of all things. As the Yang energy comes in from the outside (the sun radiating upon earth, the food we eat), it begins to move the Yin energy within, specifically at the spleen and lungs. The Yang energy causes the life force to be separated from the physical, the resulting damp mist joining up with Yin energy as it ascends to the lungs and descends into the large intestines. This separation and the coming together of Yin and Yang is the root of life and fertility, and is where infertility healing begins.

TAI YIN DISHARMONY

RECOGNIZING YOUR IMBALANCE – THE YIN ON HOLD

When an illness or blockage occurs in the Tai Yin, the Yang no longer reflects into the earth and therefore cannot stir up the Yin. Symptoms include feeling cold, fullness of abdomen, decreased appetite, loose bowels, craving for sweets, pale and thick tongue, tiredness, weak and slippery pulse, and gradual weight gain despite exercise.

CORRECTING THE IMBALANCE

DIET – STAY WITH WARM AND COOKED
Consumption of cold energy will decrease the Yang in the Tai Yin and will move you away from fertility and a healthy pregnancy. Avoid cold foods and drinks such as ice water, ice cream, or frozen desserts. Avoid water at room temperature, as well as raw fruits and vegetables.

Recommended: Beef, lamb, and slightly cooked or steamed fruits and vegetables.

HERBAL – YOUR NATURAL MORNING COCKTAIL
Add two teaspoons cinnamon powder or sticks, seven slices sun-dried ginger, one teaspoon cloves, two teaspoons sliced licorice, and one teaspoon of ginseng extract to three cups of water and boil for thirty minutes.

Drink cup after morning breakfast every day for one month.

ACUPRESSURE – BELOW THE BELT
Use fingertips to rub Stomach 36, located below the knee and one-half inch lateral to the shinbone for five minutes. Continue by

rubbing Spleen 6, located three inches above the ankle inner bone on the medial side of the leg, for five minutes. Repeat the exercise five times per day.

QI GONG — SPREAD HEAVEN'S ENERGY INTO YOUR UPPER BODY

A peaceful state of mind is crucial for success in overcoming this illness. The environment should be clean, with ample fresh air and preferably close to nature.

Wearing loose fitting clothes, and either standing or sitting down, place both hands to sides, calm the mind and regulate breathing. Close the eyes and attempt to listen inwards to the heartbeat for one minute.

Inhale deeply and exhale slowly. Raise hands above the head and stretch toward the sky. Still relaxed, imagine the hands becoming longer and longer as they reach into the heavens. Begin lowering hands, palms facing body, while imagining that heaven's energy is coming down into your head, moving down your throat, and into your chest. Place your palms on your chest and slide to lower abdomen area, heaven's energy now spreading throughout your upper body. Your palms still placed below the navale, keep your intentions and thoughts on the lower abdomen for about thirty seconds. Repeat this exercise ten times.

It is best to practice this exercise upon waking in the morning, but other times during the day will also be of benefit.

EMOTIONAL — USE MEDITATIVE HEALING TO AVOID ANGER

Avoid anger and fear as much as possible, especially over infertility issues, as these emotions damage the Tai Yin. A daily meditation just before bedtime is recommended. The meditation can be as short as one minute or as long as an hour. Begin by closing your eyes and emptying your mind. Visualize the following sentences on a big screen inside your head: "The world is constantly changing. Infertile today is fertile tomorrow. Not pregnant today is pregnant tomorrow."

LIFESTYLE – KEEP THE TEMPERATURE MODERATE AND THE AIR FRESH

Because external cold impairs the Yang from moving inwards and stirring the Yin, avoid cold temperatures caused by overactive air-conditioners at home or in the office. If nothing can be done about a cold office, dress warmly. Stay out of damp environments as much as possible, and make sure that clothes, house, vehicle and office are dry, clean, and full of fresh air.

LEVEL THREE: BUILDING A SHAO YIN RELATIONSHIP

With a Tai Yin illness, the Yang energy from the outside is unable to stir the Yin within the body. Here, in the Shao Yin, the Yang from outside the body cannot transform the Yin inside. Yang mixing with Yin is the beginning of the new life energy, the two components needed to make a baby. They interact within your body, between you and your husband and between heaven and earth. If the Yang cannot transform the Yin, conception will not occur.

RECOGNIZING THE IMBALANCE

The Shao Yin illness in your body displays itself with the following symptoms: cold hands and feet, thin weak pulse, pale white tongue. Some patients, however, manifest this illness by feeling too warm, or by feeling hot but then cold. Other patients may feel hot at night and suffer night sweats, but feel cold during the day.

REMEDYING THE IMBALANCE

DIET – BRING ON THAT CHOLESTEROL

Avoid cold food and drinks.

Include foods condensed with nutrients and energy, especially saturated fat of premium quality.

Recommended: Organic butter (preferably raw), whole nonhomogenized milk, pure cream and raw pure cheeses from grass-fed, naturally raised animals. (Availability of raw milk and cheeses varies due to state laws; visit www.realmilk.com for answers.) It is of the utmost importance that supermarket quality saturated fat not be substituted for premium quality saturated fat. It could mean the difference between success and failure.

Herbal — A potpourri for your daily use

Incorporate cinnamon, licorice, dry ginger, jujuba dates and Yin Yanghuo; remove the last leaves into teas or soups every day for one month. Bai Zhu, Sha Ren, and Cang Zhu—remove leaves; these three can also be added.

Acupressure—Use intention and imagination to bring action.

Use finger tips to massage Kidney 7 and Large Intestine 10, rubbing in energy with great intention and imagination, six times per day.

Qi Gong — Escort the life energy into your lower abdomen with your palms

Place the left palm on the center of the chest, covering the heart. Place the right palm on the lower abdomen, covering the pubic hair area. Imagine the energy emitted from the palms as filling up the chest cavity and lower abdominal cavity.

Carry out this exercise at night while lying in bed before falling asleep. Attempt to fall asleep in the same position. On waking during the night, resume the position. On waking in the morning, change to a sitting posture on the side of the bed. Place the back of the hands on the lower back, rubbing the kidney area up and down twenty-five times (up and down considered to be one rub). Breathe calmly, and slowly wake up to the new day.

EMOTIONAL: BALANCE FEAR AND JOY IN HARMONY

Avoid fear and experience joy. Fear harms the heart's ability to radiate fire. It blocks the Yang energy. Joy allows water to absorb the Yang, enabling the life force.

Fear and joy share the same root, in that they both stem from life and death. Fear is the fear of death and joy is the joy of life. In the Shao Yin sphere, fear and joy are both very necessary but must remain in balance. If in disharmony, they can harm life.

Accepting joy attracts Yang energy—the life energy of the heart. Rejecting joy blocks the Yang energy from absorption by the kidneys. Joy is the acceptance of life's energy. Fear is not the fear of failing nor is it of remaining childless. Fear is the rejection of the life force—of our fate. It is denial. It is not accepting what is happening to us. When denial is strong, or when true fear is strong, the heart's joy, expressed as fire, cannot spread and radiate to the entire body.

In the Shao Yin, the goal is to bring the joy back we experience in childhood and minimize the fear we acquire as adults. We need to dispel the fear and rid ourselves of rejection. We must stop feeling sorry for ourselves, accept our circumstances and our future. Accepting the joy frees the kidneys to spread water energy. Rejecting the fear allows the heart to spread fire energy.

LIFESTYLE MODIFICATIONS – START (OR ENHANCE) A DAILY MEDITATION PRACTICE

In Shao Yin, the interaction of water and fire is problematic. It affects the physical body, energy, emotions, and subconscious. The biggest obstacle in these two energies coming together is the distractions in our everyday lives.

When the mind is distracted, the Yang is scattered and unable to nourish the fire and water energies. We have many distractions in our life including our careers, the media, gossip, and social events. This distraction of the mind harms the Shao Yin. The reason that meditation has been so highly valued in Chinese and other

Asian cultures is because of its calming effect on the mind and the harmony that comes with it. When, by meditation, the mind is put at ease, the interaction between water and fire is facilitated.

Begin a meditation practice. If you already do practice meditation, attempt to increase the time you spend meditating. Do not keep your mind busy. Keep your mind empty.

LEVEL FOUR: BREAKING THE JUE YIN OBSTACLE

RECOGNIZING THE IMBALANCE

In the Jue Yin, the Yang wants to break apart from the Yin. A new life cycle wants to be born.

The symptoms of Jue Yin illness are thirst, a pounding heart, and hunger without the desire to eat.

CORRECTING THE IMBALANCE

DIET — EAT THAT LIVER AND ONIONS

Follow recommendations in the Tai Yin and Shao Yin sections, but in addition add organ meats (liver, heart, kidneys, brain) to your diet to strengthen the Jue Yin function of transforming the old cycle into a new one.

HERBAL

Add one teaspoon hide gelatin, thirty Goji berries, five slices dry ginger, two teaspoons cinnamon twigs, one piece ginseng, two teaspoons fennel seeds to three cups of water and boil for twenty-five minutes. Drink one cup early in morning after breakfast for one month.

ACUPRESSURE

Use left fingertips to stimulate Conception Vessel 1 (at the bottom of the trunk between the scrotum and anus), and the right palm to stimulate area of Governing Vessel 20 (top of the crown of the head).

QI GONG – BRING NATURE'S ENERGY IN

While standing, stretch both hands forward with palms open, and away from the body. Clench the fists and imagine grasping the energy in front of you. With eyes closed, take a deep breath while pulling the clenched fists to the sides of the body, then up to the chest. While doing so, imagine yourself pulling nature's energy from in front of you and into your chest cavity. Hold your breath in for five seconds while feeling the newly introduced energy in your body. With medium force, thrust your arms and hands forward, exhaling in a loud voice while abruptly opening your eyes wide. Repeat this exercise sixteen times every morning for one month.

EMOTIONAL – SOMETIMES ANGER CAN WORK

Sadness is the obstacle of Jue Yin. In a twenty-four-hour cycle, sadness begins in the evening and in an annual cycle, it begins in the fall. Nature is in decline and the Yang energy is descending.

When night comes in the daily cycle, and when winter comes in the yearly cycle, sadness ends, transforming to fear and pensiveness. Fear assists in the rejection of death and pensiveness helps to plan the next move of rebirth. If sadness fails to transform to these other emotions, the Yang life force energy in Jue Yin cannot break out and form a new cycle.

To cure this obstacle, anger is necessary. Anger is Yang energy bursting upwards. It is the opposite of sadness which drains energy. If we understand nature, we learn that each emotion has the right time as a natural and useful tool for creating and prolonging life. At the wrong time, an emotion is a destructive tool that shortens life and the ability to create it. Jue Yin needs anger, but not trivial anger over mundane things. Jue Yin needs true anger. True anger is an enormous desire to live. It is crying out loud "nobody can stop me from getting pregnant!" This is the anger needed in Jue Yin.

Since mundane anger, sadness, and resentment over trivial daily affairs are counterproductive, it is important to take actions of forgiveness and to let go of resentments. Balance the emotions in your heart.

Lifestyle modifications – A balanced exercise program

If not engaged in an exercise program already, it is time to begin. If overdoing it with exercise, now is the time to slow down. Exercise should be completed in the morning as it helps the Yang to open up. Do not go to the gym in the evening under any circumstances.

Stephanie was told that her egg quality was poor. Not ready to use egg donation, she looked for alternatives and came across the Hunyuan website. Deciding to give it a try, both Stephanie and her husband began an herbal regimen. The Hunyuan assessment by me was that the Shao Yin male-female bond was broken under the psychological pressure of the diagnosis "poor egg quality." By commencing treatment together, their problem was solved and within six months, Stephanie conceived.

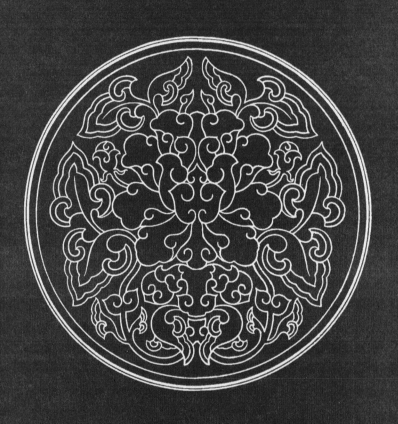

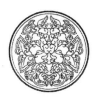

....7....

IMPROVING YOUR CHANCES
OF CONCEPTION

There are many things that couples can do to increase their chances of conception, starting with having a positive attitude.

BELIEVE IN YOURSELF

When we understand that we were created from heaven and earth and that heaven and earth are around us all the time, we can also understand that our body is capable of becoming pregnant naturally. This is what I call "Hunyuan." We all have within us this connection to heaven and earth. This connection to nature is made even before our birth and continues throughout our lives. We instinctively know how to bring the female and male energies together to create the next life. If, however, we fall into the trap of modern science, where our life is only physical and there is no heaven and earth, male and female, or Yin and Yang, then our Hunyuan is lost.

Your first step toward successful conception is to know and believe that you can do it. Believing that you can't do it, or visiting clinics that encourage you to believe that you can't do it, will harm your chances. The only question that should matter to you is how to restore a heaven-earth balance that is out of sync.

BECOME ONE WITH YOUR PARTNER

After you believe in yourself, the next most important step is to unite with your partner. To bring heaven and earth together, the husband and wife must unite. That doesn't mean you should get together to go for a consultation at the IVF clinic. Rather, it means that you must be in it together all the way from beginning to end. Disharmony of heaven and earth is always a disharmony of the male and female. In contrast to modern medicine, which pinpoints the blame on the wife or the husband, in Chinese medicine it is always the couple's disharmony that needs to be restored. "Getting pregnant" is a man and woman coming together and "infertility" is a man and a woman who can't come together.

Although the remedies given to men and women may be different, the goal of the mutual remedy is to allow their unification. Otherwise, the unification is broken, and a new relationship begins; doctor-wife or doctor-husband. The intervention of the doctor between husband and wife does not exist with Chinese medicine. With IVF, for example, the doctor assumes the role of the husband, intervening at the time of conception by delivering the sperm to the egg. The male heaven is not there, even if his sperm is. The time of the Jue Yin is fragile and delicate, and it needs the perfect harmony of heaven and earth to allow the Yin to close and to allow the Yang to be born. Instead, the physician intrudes into the female body, creating great difficulty.

If the husband and wife are healthy, then heaven and earth come together in harmony. During the course of treatment, it is important for me to locate the disharmony with the husband as it relates to his wife, and the disharmony with the wife as it relates to her husband; then both husband and wife receive the necessary herbs to correct this disharmony. Each herbal formula aims at harmonizing the couple by bringing them closer to each other. Every couple's situation is different and while sometimes I use only herbs for both partners, sometimes I also use acupuncture for the wife, because the female is Yin and acupuncture can bring the Yin outside to meet the Yang. These treatments bring the couple back into harmony and enable them to conceive.

EXERCISE THE RIGHT WAY

The goal of exercising is to restore and improve health. It is not to burn calories or to lose weight. While trying to get pregnant and after you are pregnant, it is particularly important to exercise in a sensible way. The guiding principle for exercise is to avoid doing too much or too little.

Exercise should be done gently with minimum impact on the body. Overstraining the muscles and ligaments is not healthy. High impact exercises should be avoided as they damage the joints and tendons, which in turn will cause the liver to deteriorate (the liver nourishes the tendons and will be overtaxed). The liver is the first organ to support the embryo, and if the liver is weak, the embryo will not develop or will not implant. Heavy perspiration during exercise and exhaustion of the muscles will cause the spleen to deteriorate; it is the spleen that nourishes the muscles. If the spleen is tired, the Yang energy cannot rise in the body and a pregnancy cannot stick. Unlike heavy impact exercises, light exercise stimulates the tendons and muscles by encouraging the liver and spleen to circulate energy. This in turn will improve fertility and pregnancy.

To tell whether your exercise regimen is too heavy or too light, pay attention to your body and the way you are feeling. Heavy sweat, sore muscles, and achy joints are indications of too much exercise. Not perspiring at all, stiff joints, and no feeling of an increase in energy indicates a lack of exercise.

Tai Chi and Yoga, which are more body-friendly, involve learning breathing and relaxation tecŸiques that can improve the body, energy, and spirit. These disciplines are beneficial when it comes to trying to conceive as well as during pregnancy. It is important to find an experienced teacher who can guide you through.

TIMING CONCEPTION – OPEN YOUR OWN WINDOW

Every woman has a window of fertility in the middle of the menstrual cycle which lasts approximately ten days. This window can shift depending on the length of the cycle. In a regular twenty-eight-day cycle, it is from days nine to nineteen. In a short menstrual cycle of twenty-four days, it is from days five to fifteen. In a long menstrual cycle of forty days, it is from days twenty-one to thirty-one.

To calculate your fertility window, take the number of days of your last menstrual cycle and subtract fourteen to reach your mid-fertile point, the middle of the window. Then subtract five from the mid-fertile point to pinpoint the window's first day, the first day to begin having intercourse. From the mid-fertile point, add five days to identify the last day of the window, when intercourse should stop.

In our example, if the last menstrual cycle is twenty-eight days, the mid-fertile point is day fourteen of the cycle, the beginning day for intercourse is day nine, and the end day of the fertile window is day nineteen. Let's say that the last menstrual cycle is forty days long, the mid-fertile day is day twenty-six (40-14=26), the beginning day is day twenty-one (26-5=21), and the end day is day thirty-one (26+5=31).

This calculation method is only good for women who have a regular cycle. If the cycle is irregular, modern tecŸiques of detecting ovulation will be necessary.

BEST TIME FOR INTERCOURSE – DON'T DEPLETE THE HUBBY

Once you have established your fertile window, knowing how to optimize that time is the next step. Contrary to what some people might think, daily intercourse during your fertile window will not improve your chances of getting pregnant. It will actually decrease your chances, as daily intercourse will deplete your husband's resources. You should establish a rhythm of one intercourse session every other day.

The time of day will also have an effect on your chances of conceiving. The best chances for conception come with intercourse that occurs in the morning, the time that the body is most rested and when the Yang energy opens up to become more active. The Jue Yin, when the Yin comes to extinction and the new Yang is born, extends from 1 A.M. to 7 A.M. It is a time of "war" between Yin and Yang, when the liver, which is the Jue Yin organ, is the "general" who calls the decisions. Even when intercourse occurs at 4 P.M. the prior day, conception and implantation will occur during Jue Yin time in the early morning hours.

COMMON MISTAKES AND HOW TO AVOID THEM

In modern medicine, conception is often viewed as a mechanical event: The egg meets the sperm and they create an embryo. When we follow this line of thinking, then timing the ovulation is the essence of fertility treatments. However, in Chinese medicine, conception involves many more factors such as the heaven and earth and the male and female energies. When the energies are aligned correctly, then the egg and sperm will perform their natural function with ease. We are therefore most concerned with disturbances to energy, mind, and spirit.

Most common modern recommendations to time ovulation are not only ineffective but also counterproductive. Ovulation kits and measuring basal body temperatures increase the female and male anxiety and thus create energy obstructions. When the woman anxiously awaits ovulation, she transmits this anxiety to her male partner, the liver energy becomes stagnant, and the Jue Yin suffers. When the Jue Yin can't break apart the Yin and Yang, then conception cannot happen. The "general" is restrained and can't lead this war into a victory.

Using the fertility calculation above is preferable to ovulation kits because it does not involve stress and anxiety. The only exception is when the menstrual cycle is very irregular and must first be regulated in order to detect the fertile window.

More than knowing the fertility window is necessary for conception. Many myths have developed around intercourse and conception. These myths often propagate incorrect or counterproductive methods and can interfere with a couple's ability to conceive. One common myth is the notion that couples should attempt to have intercourse in a variety of strange positions. The path to successful conception is the natural way, with heaven on top and earth below, meaning the man is on top and the female is below.

Another common myth is that the woman should lie in bed for a period of time after intercourse. This is false. When the female stands up, the vertical line inside her uterus becomes horizontal. We call the vertical line, which connects heaven and earth, Jing. When the woman stands, the newly formed embryo has changed its position from horizontal to vertical, or from Wei to Jing. The newly conceived life has just changed from a lifeless pre-heaven state to a post-heaven state that is full of life.

The father on top and the mother below can make this pre-heaven vertical (Jing) line inside the uterus prepare for conception. Thereafter the mother changes position and stands up so the embryo has its first change from Jing to Wei, from vertical to horizontal. Although in the modern era, men and women have intercourse in a variety of positions, the traditional position is lying down with the male on top and the female below. This is because it is the energetic state needed for conception.

Patients often tell me that through online research they have come upon four requirements for successful conception: staying in bed after intercourse, placing a pillow under the hips during sex, elevating the feet in the air immediately thereafter, and not bathing or showering for at least one day. None of these actions will have any affect whatsoever on fertility.

YOUR BABY IS WHAT YOU EAT

Prior to visiting my office, a thirty-nine-year-old patient had conceived naturally. Unfortunately, an ectopic pregnancy resulted, requiring the fallopian tube to be removed. Thereafter, the patient became convinced that IVF would be her only option. Even though IVF does not eliminate the possibility for an ectopic pregnancy, it does nevertheless decrease its probability.

After two failed IVFs, I recommended to the patient that she try an herbal course. The patient politely declined while stating the following reason: "I had a DES exposure while in my mother's womb, and because of that, I am certain that only IVF will be appropriate."

Why am I bringing up this story? Because I believe it characterizes our entire modern society. Although her mother used artificial hormones that actually caused the patient's problem, the patient was still confident that using modern hormones and drugs today would have no negative impact on her baby in the future.

To expand on the importance of parental choices with regard to the health of their offspring, let us turn to a book by a prominent gynecologist from the Qing Dynasty (1644-1911), Zhang Yao Sun's *Pregnancies, Labor and Delivery Collections*. In Chapter Three, *Appropriate Actions During Pregnancy*, he wrote: "When the baby lives in his mother's womb, the mother's Qi is his Qi, the mother's blood is his blood and the mother's breath is his breath. When the mother's heart is virtuous, her Qi and blood harmonize well and the baby will grow to be of great health. When the mother's heart is poor, her Qi and blood are in chaos and the baby will suffer. It is important to remember that the mother's Qi being pure or turbid, or her heart being virtuous or poor, are all affected by the seasons and everything else with which she comes in contact.

"The Qi is controlled by the heart. The heart's spirit rules the interior of the body and it reacts to the exterior. Whenever the body comes in contact with the exterior, the spirit moves and the Qi follows. When the mother comes in contact with 'Virtuous,' the Yang energy moves and the Qi becomes pure. When she comes in contact with 'Poor,' the Yin energy moves and the Qi becomes turbid. Because of that, the pregnant woman must be cautious of what she comes in contact with. As soon as the baby is conceived, it digests myriad things. These myriad things are all what the mother ingests and digests. In ancient times, the pregnant woman will not lay or sit in an awkward place, she will not ingest any evil flavors, she will not eat anything which is not by nature. Oh! Pregnant woman, know that you can teach your fetus to become like a king or to become a beautiful nobleman."

It is for every woman to consider what she injects into her bloodstream in terms of how it will impact her baby. As Confucius said: "Only doing it before is wisdom, while doing it after is foolish. The reason for that is before birth, the truth, even tiny, already manifests itself, and the affair seems small but it is actually grand. For the heart of the knowledgeable person knows the truth and so he makes changes in his life accordingly." Making your child healthy after he is born cannot equal making your child healthy before he is born.

Susie and Stephen could not conceive. Deciding that drugs and IVF treatments were not for them, they grew convinced that the best approach was to become healthy first. They reached out to me and the Hunyuan Method, and within thirty days conceived naturally.

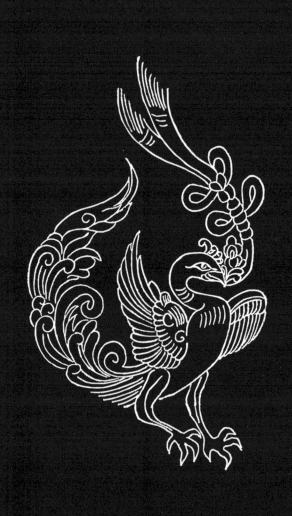

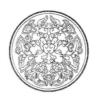

····8····

CULTURE GIVES BIRTH TO MEDICINE

A visitor called, clad in his best robes, and awaited the arrival of his host in the reception room. A rat, which had been disporting itself upon the beams above, insinuating its nose into a jar of oil which was put there for safekeeping,, became frightened at the sudden intrusion of the caller. It ran away, and in so doing upset the oil jar, which fell directly on the caller, striking him a severe blow and ruining his elegant garments.

Just as the face of the guest was purple with rage at this disaster, the host entered. When the proper salutations were performed, the guest proceeded to explain the situation, "As I entered your honorable apartment and seated myself under your honorable beam, I inadvertently terrified your honorable rat, which fled and upset your honorable oil jar upon my mean and insignificant clothing, which is the reason for my contemptible appearance in your honorable presence."

This is a story told by the Swedish sinologist and philologist Bernard Kalgren (1889–1978) to describe a culture fundamentally different than ours in the West. It is a culture rooted with moral values dating back 4,500 years where a guest must always esteem his host and humble himself, regardless of the circumstances.

The medicine sage Sun Simiao in the seventh century AD wrote in his book Emergency Prescriptions Worth a Thousand Gold: *"To have Da Yi (great physician or great medicine), one must be versed with the ancient classics. Why is this so? Because if one does not know the five classics, he will never know virtue and compassion." The texts known as The Confucius Classics for the past 2,500 years, because they were compiled and edited by Confucius at the age of forty-three, are:* Yi Jing (Book of Changes), Liji (Book of Rites), Shiji (Book of Odes), Shujing (The Book), Chunqiu (Spring and Autumn Annals).

For us Westerners, to understand the intrinsic value of Chinese medicine, we need to understand the fertile soil out of which it grows. As with the story we just read, why would an angry man call his host repeatedly "honorable" even when he is furious? The "Confucius classics," dealing with such questions, were edited and compiled in the sixth century BC; however, the information written in them dates back as far as the Xia and Shang dynasties (twenty-fourth century BC–twelfth century BC).

Chinese culture was rich in social morals and behaviors back as far as 4,000 years ago. The Chinese written language developed as a language of symbols. First, it was an ancient script on oracle bones used for imperial divination, and later on it was a sophisticated system of symbols used by the common people.

The ancients used symbols to reach for the why's and what's of life. The famous physician Zhang Jingyue (1563–1640 AD) in his book *Additions to Lei Jing* wrote, "Medicine equals the art of symbols. It contains the complexity of Yin Yang movement and stillness. Medicine equals the art of ideas. It joins with the Yin Yang mechanism of growth and decline. Even though *The Yellow Emperor* classic talks about Yin and Yang, there is nothing greater than the book of changes. It is said that heaven and earth unite into one principle of Yin and Yang. *The Changes* (Yi) and medicine share a common origin, both dwell in the research of transformation. They are interchangeably dependent and their philosophies join as one. How can you become a doctor, then, and not know *The Changes* (Yi)?

In our lifetime, the Yin and Yang are in constant change. The Jing-Wei and Xing-Ming are constant; however, the time elapsing every day, every season, and every year carry a different weight, transforming our life into an active ever-changing situation. What we strive for with medicine is to understand the weight in between the fixed positions in order to establish the correct weight for harmony. Chinese medicine is not the study of static Yin and Yang, it is rather the study of the weight influencing Yin and Yang. Yin and Yang are visible; however, the transformation of the two is not. I can see the day and I can see the night, but I cannot see the change in between. I can see a live person and I can see a dead person, but I cannot see the change between the phases.

The same goes for fertility, conception, and pregnancy. We can see the situation before the baby is conceived, namely the father and mother having intercourse. The baby's Yin and Yang are static. The Yang from the father is separated from the Yin of the mother. In other words, there is no embryo yet. Setting aside unnatural modern medicine procedures and equipment, we can see the baby after it comes out to the world, but we cannot see the development of the baby inside the abdomen of the woman. The post-heaven trigrams represent the life of the baby after it is born. For the rest of its life, changes will occur constantly until death. In between the two pre-heaven and post-heaven scenarios, we have the "change." This change is conception and pregnancy, the unification of the father and mother into a new life. It is the invisible change we cannot see with our eyes, yet we can measure its weight and meanings with symbols and numbers.

If we think about conception, the male has only one option. He can only give his sperm to the female. His steps go in one direction. The female has two options. She can go underneath with all steps in one direction, thus aiming at giving her essence/egg to the male. On the other hand, she can open up and cross underneath and above at the same time. This allows her to receive the male sperm, meaning that a female can choose, by her actions, if she wants to receive the male essence or not. If she moves in one direction she behaves like the male and at this time, conception is not possible. If she opens herself up to move in two opposite directions, she behaves like a female and unification can happen, creating a new life. This is why a Yin line is a broken line. It can open up in two directions. The Yang is only one line and it can move in one direction.

The earth is the mother of the myriad things. The earth can be fertile or infertile. It depends on how receptive it is to the heaven Yang. If the earth receives the heavenly Yang, life will grow out of it. Important to understand from this image is that the male has no choice, but the female does. If a female acts as Yang, then conception is difficult, but if she acts as Yin, conception is easy. It carries meaning on many different levels and each woman should self-examine and decide what more can she do to become Yin. One thing

Natalie and Bob were hoping to get pregnant immediately after their wedding, but it failed to happen for a year. They decided against pursuing the path of drugs and invasive tests. Health conscious and consumers of organic foods, they were concerned about the possible side effects drugs might have on their baby. Natalie had been told that she was infertile because her mother used a drug while pregnant with her and Natalie had promised not to make the same mistake with her own child. Natalie and Bob found the Hunyuan Method through a friend and after six months of herbs and acupuncture, they conceived naturally. They gave birth to a healthy baby who reportedly became the smartest boy in his class!

is clear according to the classics, a man needs to be a gentleman, caring, protecting, and nourishing the woman. A woman does not necessarily need to be a gentleman. When we compare the images of the steps, we can also see that the male goes from one side to the other or from inside out. In contrast, the female goes to the other side and comes back. This is a clear distinction between Yin and Yang behavior. This is why, during intercourse, the male can give to the female, but the female cannot give to the male. The Yin action is to take in, while the Yang action is to give out. These Yin and Yang steps are conception and pregnancy. They are the change connecting the pre-heaven (before conception/ perfect balance) to the post-heaven (life/ constant change of Yin-Yang seven, eleven).

The science of symbols and numbers allowing us to understand life is the tool that can help us understand Chinese medicine better and in return solve infertility more successfully. Answers to very difficult questions not answered by modern science may be answered. For example, why does a woman produce one egg per menstrual cycle, while a man produces 100 million sperm with each ejaculation? Why, when a man produces so many millions of sperm, only one sperm makes it to the egg? Why does one sperm plus one egg make only one baby?

CONCLUSION

Medicine is medicine. As I've stated previously in this book, there is no Chinese medicine or Western medicine, there is only good or bad medicine. Chen Xiuyuan says, "Medicine is in the hands of the doctor and not in the hands of the profession."

A prospective father came to me with maturation arrest and zero sperm count. I recommended herbs, but his doctor was opposed, claiming herbs as "not being scientific" and further insisting that it might impact his hormones and make things worse. I explained to the patient that there is nothing worse than zero. He was still

223

worried, and for four months, commenced rigorous medical tests, preparing for sperm extraction from his testicles. At the same time, he decided to try Chinese herbs. To his excitement and the doctor's surprise, within sixty days, sperm began appearing in his semen and extraction was avoided.

Another patient, diagnosed with blood clotting disorder, suffered six miscarriages while trying different blood thinning medications to no avail. After two months of herbs and acupuncture, she began carrying a perfectly healthy baby to term. No blood thinning herbs were used, only herbs supporting the Yang.

The challenge of medicine is with the eyes of the doctor. In classical Chinese medicine we recognize high - and low-level practitioners. High-level practitioners see a different method and recognize its strong points, while low-level practitioners see its deficiencies. The one who sees the other's strong points can coexist and thrive, while the one who sees the weak points will always be separated, rivaled and short lived. Western medicine has many strong points, mainly its expertise in the physical body. Chinese medicine has strong points, mainly its expertise in life. The body belongs to earth, while life belongs to heaven. If heaven and earth are separated, it is the pre-heaven scenario. There is no life. However, if heaven and earth, each doing its own job, are connected, then life thrives.

Heaven needs to act like heaven and earth needs to act like earth. Heaven and earth connected together does not mean that heaven behaves like earth, rather, it means that they are joined together in harmony. Chinese medicine is medicine of heaven and time. Western medicine is medicine of earth and space. When the two medicines join together it is the best that can happen to our bodies and to our lives.

I believe that the future of medicine is in the hands of high-level practitioners of east and west who recognize the strong points on the other side because, in their hearts, they truly care about their patients. Medicine is here to help and heal people, to prolong lives, and to ensure the well-being of future generations. It must learn from the past and look to the future.

It is time to go back to classical thinking. It is time for a change. In the West, the doctor should know patients personally and treat them as if they were his own family as it used to be in the last 2,000 years. In the East, practitioners should read the classics again, understand more about life and leave Western medicine for Western doctors. Joining forces so our kids can grow up healthy is the moral calling of the healer. The patient needs to know it. The doctor needs to know it. Officials and policy makers need to follow along.

Healing life is an art, while fixing the body is tecŸology. It is like a piano and music, they are both important. The same is true with medicine. The one who can fix the muscles and bones is as important as the one who can fix the life force. For the sake of patients and future generations, both need to be available to our society.

Infertility patients often talk about "window of opportunities closing down." This brings to my mind a folk song I knew as a little boy:

> Open the gate, open it wide
> through it there shall pass a golden thread;
> mother, father, sister and brother
> bride and a groom in a chariot of life.
> Open the gate, open it wide
> through it there shall pass a golden thread;
> grandpa and grandma, uncle and aunt
> grandchildren and great-grandchildren
> in a chariot of strung pearls
> Open the gate, open it wide.

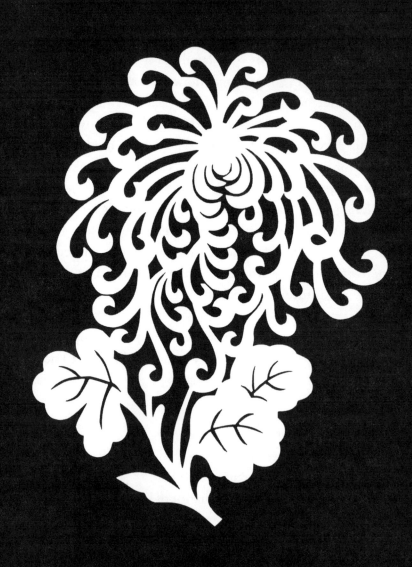

APPENDIX A – PATIENT TESTIMONIALS

Dear Dr. Seidman,

We want to thank you for giving us the most special gift—our little daughter I.M. After countless fertility treatments, failed IVF procedures, and tearful doctor consultations, we were about to give up on conceiving. We turned to you as a last resort, after our doctor recommended using an egg donor, which is a path we did not want to take. I was very skeptical at first at the thought of taking herbs and doing acupuncture to help my fertility. How can something so simple help me to conceive? But after only two months under your care, I was pregnant!! We were so surprised, and so thrilled.

Unfortunately, we found you after we had spent thousands of dollars on fertility treatments. If only we had gone to you sooner. We now have a beautiful, healthy little girl. She is now six weeks old, and changing every day. Sometimes when I look at her, I'm filled with such emotion. My husband and I are so thankful to have her in our lives. We truly believe that it was your treatments that brought us to a successful pregnancy.

Thank you so much, and good luck with your own baby to be!

Regards, C. & D.

Dr. Seidman,

I am sorry we have not been by to visit again. We think and speak often about you—you are one of our favorite people.

Speaking of favorite people, here is another. (Look carefully.. two little pearly whites have popped up!

Warmly, C.

Dear Dr. Seidman,

Thank you very much for all of your help. The herbal treatments and the acupuncture helped me so much. The treatments helped me to get pregnant and I felt strong and healthy again. In February we were blessed with the birth of our healthy daughter L. She has brought us so much joy and happiness. We are so grateful to you—your kindness and care are much appreciated.

L.

Dear Dr. Seidman,

There are no words to describe how grateful we are for all the help in making our dream come true! A. is a very content, happy and healthy child, much loved by her brother.

Truly, C.F.

Dear Dr. Seidman,

Our daughter, A. will turn one in August. Thank you for helping us bring her about.

You probably recall that my husband was very skeptical about trying herbs, but that I had watched peers undergo what I consider invasive measures unsuccessfully. I kept hearing that, in the end, herbs and acupuncture had the best results. At age forty-two, I did not want to waste a whole year or more on Western medicine, only to be disappointed.

My pregnancy was typical and the delivery was without incident. A, arrived one day after the predicted date.

Again, we thank you and wish good things for others under your care.

N.B.

Dear Dr. Seidman,

Thank you so much for all your help. I am very happy to report M. is growing very healthy and rapidly. She is almost six weeks old now. Thankfully, your herbs and acupuncture got me pregnant. Thank you again. When I am ready to try for the baby number two, I will call you again!

M.C.

Dear Dr. Seidman,

I would have never thought I would be able to get pregnant. Three years ago, I suffered from a stroke. My right side was numb and I suffered terrible back pains. Two years of physio didn't help.

Trying to get pregnant of course didn't work either. The doctors kept me on blood thinners that made it very difficult for me to get pregnant. I have started acupuncture and herbal treatment and after four months the back pains were gone and my right side felt as if I had never had a stroke.

When you asked me if I was planning to get pregnant, I was convinced that there was nothing you could do to help me. I took herbs for four more months, I got pregnant and my baby is nine months old today. My life has changed completely since I came for the first time to your office.

I am grateful forever.

T.

Dear Dr. Seidman,

Almost four years ago I suffered a miscarriage which was devastating. My husband and I tried unsuccessfully to conceive again and after a year of trying we went to a fertility specialist.

We went through two years of tests, endless needles, blood work, medications, 6 failed artificial inseminations and two failed IVF cycles. Every Doctor we went to said everything looked "normal" and we should keep trying different protocols. Not one Doctor could give us a reason as to why I could produce eggs but not fertilize them. One IVF cycle I produced twenty-nine eggs and not one took. All they could tell me was because of my age it is more difficult, I was thirty-six years old.

Needless to say those years were filled with many tears. Tears of sorrow and frustration. A friend recommended you to me and I thought I would give a more natural course a try. I was a little skeptical to be quite honest, but I figured if nothing else, I could detoxify myself from the past years worth of infertility drugs I had taken.

From our first visit in April 2003 you told me straight on exactly why I could not get pregnant. I thought, "Finally, someone is giving me a solid reason." The beautiful part was that there were no painful needles or intrusive exams.

After three months of being on your prescribed herbs, and twenty days of my husband being on herbs, we conceived in August 2003. I am thrilled to tell you we gave birth in April to a beautiful healthy baby boy.

Doctor Seidman, thank you. Thank you for always answering all my questions, being straight forward with me and giving me the answers I was searching for. More importantly thank you for our son!

Sincerely, M.

Dear Dr. Seidman,

I wanted to share my story with other patients who consider your services. I have been taking herbs for six months, and while I did not get pregnant I went to a reproductive endocrinologist to try IVF. The RE told me at the 3rd day blood test that my FSH was high—twenty-eight—so I was disqualified for the IVF. He suggested I use a donor egg. To my amazement, this same month we conceived naturally. I was sure I'll miscarry, but I am twenty-five weeks now and everything seems great. I am so thankful for your help, as this could have never happened without you.

D.S.

Dear Dr. Seidman,

I am writing this letter to help other women who find themselves in a position I once was. I had problems getting pregnant for 2 years. I have tried Clomaid and three artificial inseminations. Eventually I had no choice but to go through an IVF procedure. Not only I did not get pregnant, my reproductive endocrinologist advised me that a future IVF will not work, and that I should look into a Donor Egg.

You see, I have only produced one egg of poor quality and my progesterone levels were not right. I have started my herbal treatment, and even though it was a bitter tea I have never tasted before, I persisted.

Guess what? It was five months later that I found out to my amaze that I am fifth week pregnant. I found out while I was on a trip to St. Louis. I am not sure if you were able in Connecticut to hear me screaming (of joy) all the way from there.

There are only two words I can summarize my experience with: Thank You.

J.

Dear Dr. Seidman,

I just wanted to send you a note to THANK YOU! for your help in bringing E. to us. There is no way for us to adequately express our appreciation. Here is a picture at four weeks old!

Love,

J. & M.

Hi Dr. Seidman,

How are you? I just took two pregnancy tests today and both results were positive that I am pregnant. Could the herbs be affecting the results?

I am going to get a blood test tomorrow at my OB/GYN. I am really surprised right now to say the least!

Thanks, S.B.

Dear Dr. Seidman,

I wanted to ask if the herbs could affect a pregnancy test. I drank half a cup on Wednesday night. I took the pregnancy test on Thursday night, but I didn't take the herbs that night. The test was positive. I tested again early this morning and it is positive.

Let me know what you think.

Am I really pregnant?

D.

Dear Dr. Seidman,

Hi, hope you are well. I got back my positive results & had an Ultrasound to confirm I am pregnant. You have been so amazing to me and have helped me out so much. I really appreciate everything you have done for me. Thank you so much.

Sincerely, S.

Hi Dr. Seidman,

I can't believe it I had yesterday only three follicles, and after having one acupuncture session I went in for ultrasound today and we saw six. After a week of stimming and no response, the doctor just doesn't know where these follicles came from all of a sudden. I guess we will go to retrieval after all.

Thanks a million, D.

Dear Dr. Seidman,

Your reading of my pulse was right. It turned out I am pregnant and thrilled. I couldn't believe when you said the pulse looked pregnant, but amazingly it is true.

Wow.

M.

Dr. Seidman,

We are so grateful to you for all the help you gave us. We feel so fortunate to have our son in our lives now. Your attention and care were so appreciated. We believed in making a difference and achieving success. We hope you can meet our son soon. With great thanks,

J. & S.

Dear Dr. Seidman,

I had never had very regular periods, but at age twenty-six, my periods stopped altogether. I was hoping to get pregnant in the near future and asked my OB/GYN about my chances. She referred me to a Reproductive Endocrinologist (RE) who diagnosed me with low estrogen levels. My RE recommended using injectable fertility drugs to get pregnant. I didn't see any other way, so I decided to give it a try even though my health insurance didn't cover the cost of the treatment. I went through two injectable cycles, one IUI and the other IVF, resulting in a chemical pregnancy and a miscarriage, respectively. In only a few months, I had gained fifteen pounds from the hormones and spent over $15,000 with nothing but heartache as a result.

It was at this point that I read about the use of acupuncture and Chinese herbs as infertility treatments. I decided that I had nothing to lose and gave the Hunyuan center a call. I was skeptical of the Hunyuan method, but I decided to have some faith and give the herbs a chance. After a month and a half, I had light spotting and was encouraged. A little over a month later, I was pregnant. I couldn't believe it was so easy after all that we have been through. I had acupuncture treatments during my first trimester to help prevent a miscarriage, and they really helped me relax. I gave birth to a beautiful, healthy baby girl who is one of the most easygoing and happy babies I have ever seen. I can't be thankful enough for this joy.

J.

Dr. Seidman,

Thank you from the bottom of our hearts for all your help and support.

K.

Dr. Seidman,

An amazing thing happened W. did not get her period, and did a pregnancy test which came up with a second line indicating she may be pregnant. It was a faint line but it was definitely there and she never ever had one before, and she checks herself every month. We are going to repeat the test tomorrow.

She did not drink tea tonight and we wanted to know if she should continue with it. Please email me tomorrow. Also we wanted to continue with treatments even if she is pregnant. And need to know about your post conception programs. I look forward to your email.

Thank you for all your help.

Best Regards,

J.

Dear Dr. Seidman,

It has been an amazing two years since the birth of our beautiful baby girl, S. She is truly a blessing to our family and we are so very grateful to you for your assistance in bringing her into our lives. My husband and I were trying for over a year to get pregnant and were unsuccessful. We tried various traditional infertility options and stopped just before beginning more intensive treatments. I was fortunate enough to learn about your method through another success story patient who told me about it. I am so glad that we gave the Hunyuan Method a try before going to intramuscular injections, etc, both because I was not looking forward to the pain of those shots and because after only being on herbs for one month, we learned that we were pregnant! It was so simple, painless and natural. Not only were you able to help us get pregnant, but you also brought me to a stronger sense of health and well-being in general. I would (and have!) tell anyone in this situation to give the Hunyuan Method a try. Centuries of successful pregnancies can't be wrong! Here is a picture of our little one..thank you, thank you, thank you!

All the best, T.

Hi Dr. Seidman,

Hope all is well. Over the past two weeks, I lost track of time with scheduling an appointment. Yesterday, to our great disbelief, after being five days late, I took a home pregnancy test and it was positive! We are proceeding very cautiously and I am going for a blood test today. Interestingly, a blood test on Day Twenty-One led the doctor to believe that my estrogen and progesterone were 'normal' but that I was probably not pregnant. So we are bit mystified.

Thanks so much, P.

Dr. Seidman,

Words can't express my gratitude to you. I know that the acupuncture was a big help in conceiving this beautiful baby. But even more important was your caring nature. You helped me to believe that I would have a baby and taught me patience. Thank you so very much for everything. We are enjoying these early days with C. and will come by soon to visit you.

M.K.

Dr. Seidman:

Our story is a bit less complex than most of your patients, but surely others can relate. As you know, I faced issues relating to pregnancy as I had a history of miscarriages. After having a third miscarriage, my gynecologist recommended my husband and I make an appointment to discuss infertility options with an infertility clinic. At the time I was thirty-two years old and thought there had to be a better way. I ended up finding you by chance as I was researching options. At first, I was not too sure how you would help. But after I began to understand the Hunyuan Method I was less skeptical and trusted in your method. After six months of following your direction and taking the herbs specific for my needs, we did in fact become pregnant again. This time, however, we stayed pregnant! Our little girl, K. R., is now ten months old. Like most that have experienced having a child, I look at her and think of how blessed we are to share our lives together. From time to time I also think of how blessed I was to find you and trust in your expertise as you helped to make this experience possible. Thank you Dr. Seidman.

C.

Hi Dr. Seidman,

I just wanted to let you know that our new little girl has arrived! Her name is P.L. and we call her P. for short. She was born on Sunday, August 26 at 7:43 P.M. and she weighed in at 6 lbs. 12 ounces. She is a delight – mom and dad are both thrilled! Thank you so much for everything that you have done for our family. I have already recommended you to other friends of mine who are struggling to build a family and if we decide that we would like a second child, we will be back!

Thank you again – my husband, P. and I are all so grateful to have had you as our doctor.

Warmly, A.F.

Dr. Seidman,

Once again – thank you very much for all your help and support (the second baby with Hunyuan). T.

Dear Dr. Seidman,

M. is born Saturday the 29th at 2h56 am: 7 pounds and 20 inches.

So far she is in perfect health. I keep thinking "thanks to Dr Seidman".

We're so happy of her. She's alert and yet serene. And of course she's the most beautiful baby in the world!

To go on with the good health we would like to come and begin with the breastfeeding plan.

Yours, C.

It seems the fifth time was the charm! Our son J. T. was born last Tuesday, 7 lbs., 10 oz.

Thanks so much for your work with us. We greatly appreciated your effort and understanding.

So, best wishes to you and thanks.

G.K.

Hi Dr. Seidman,

I have been meaning to e-mail you lately. Hope you and your family are well and that your son is growing leaps and bounds! Our little girl surprised us and decided she wanted to come early! I will send you a picture and stop by someday soon. I can't tell how grateful we are to you. Each time she opens her beautiful eyes and looks at us, J. and I well up with joy and know that she wouldn't be here if we had not found you.

Hope to see you soon, P.B.

Hi Dr. Seidman-

Well, it happened early – I gave birth to J.W. in November. He's doing great...

I don't think I'll be leaving the house for the next few months, so I'll start again next year when we're ready to try for another one!!

Thanks again for all your help with this pregnancy. I truly believe that you are the reason I finally got pregnant and had a healthy baby boy!! You are a sensational healer. I'll send pictures soon.

A.W.

Hello Dr. Seidman,

I just wanted to send you an update – I am SEVENTEEN weeks pregnant and all looks good. We had our triple screen with the nuchal ultrasound and the baby is fine. I also started feeling the baby move this week! Our due date is ~ May 28th.

Thank you again for all of your help!

Enjoy the holidays,

J.

Hi Yaron-

I just got off the phone with a friend who made an appointment with you on Saturday. Their struggle with infertility is similar to mine, but they already have one child. I am hopeful that you will be able to help them, because to me you are a miracle worker. Their names are A. and D. Good luck! I'm really excited they finally decided to come talk to you!

Things here are going well. Little N. is thriving and putting on good weight. Having a child is harder than I thought though, I must admit. I attached a picture of my dog and N. for you.

I'll try and stop in sometime soon with N. so you can meet your creation.

Hope things are going well.

Thanks, A.

Yaron,

We are extraordinarily grateful for your help and care, without which I am certain we wouldn't have G. He is heaven-sent! Your work is superb.

K.

Dear Dr. Seidman,

We are sending you THANK YOUS! galore. Here is a picture of our two miracles that you helped bring to us. Everyone is doing well. Thank you seems such a small way to express our gratitude for walking with us through this journey. We can never fully express all that you have done for us. Your family will always be in our prayers!

Love J., M., E. and M.

Hi Dr. Seidman!

It's been a while since we last "spoke!" I hope you are doing well! Everything with me is going really well. I am writing for a couple of reasons:

(1) The biggest news of all... WE'RE PREGNANT!!!!!!!!! Yes, it's true! Can you believe it? I am in my thirteenth week, and feeling very good. I want to thank you because I think you had a lot to do with it! We conceived in early April, and I know that the effects of acupuncture/herbs can last for several months. So, THANK YOU! It is truly our dream come true! We feel so very blessed. Life seems all new now! What a wonderful, welcome surprise!

(2) I also wanted to see if acupuncture is indicated during pregnancy. If so, I would like to set up a couple of appointments by the end of the month. Would you have any appointments available? Please let me know.

And thank you, thank you, thank you once again! I look forward to seeing you soon!

All the best, D.

Dear Dr. Seidman:

As I told you this morning, I went to see the doctor today for an ultrasound. I remembered that you had said in all your successes you have never had twins before. Well, there is a first time for everything. The ultrasound showed twins today. It is still too early to say whether I will deliver twins but the doctor seemed pretty confident that both babies had strong heartbeats. Let's keep our fingers crossed and doing what we are doing.

I'll see you on Sat.
D.

I started working with Dr. Seidman and doing herbal therapy because we wanted to have one more successful pregnancy. In addition to trying to get pregnant, I had several other conditions I was dealing with. I had Chronic Lyme disease and had undergone an extensive oral and IV antibiotic treatment for a total of four years. The treatment left my digestive system very weak and I had chronic fatigue. I was also older and a neurotic nervous wreck as a result of the fertility tests and the miscarriages and I felt time was running out.

Despite it all, I persisted with the herbs, and finally, we had our little baby. I was forty-three years old.

Writing this letter allows me the opportunity to share some of my life experiences with those who are going through similar challenges, and also to say thank you to Dr. Seidman for helping me accomplish great things in my life.
M.

Dr. Seidman,

I just wanted to share some great news with you. If you remember our story, we did a number of IUIs and IVFs over the past few years. They all failed and doctors did not seem to have an explanation for it. My husband and I met with you last October and by December I was pregnant. On August 11th we welcomed a beautiful very healthy happy little boy! We named him A. R. We thank you for making our dream come true. His birth was very emotional for us. We continue to tell all our friends, family members and coworkers about you and your website. We will be back to you for our next one when we are ready! We have included a picture of our miracle! Thanks again!

L. and C.

APPENDIX B – THE ZODIAC SIGNS

The Chinese sages used a system of twelve zodiac signs, referred to as "the twelve earthly branches," to draw parallels in assimilating the time concept of today and tomorrow. While the twenty-four Qi explain how to break down Yin and Yang into pieces, the twelve zodiac signs show you how to unify the entire time concept into one. They also created ten "heavenly stems," a system of ten zodiac signs to describe heaven's energy.

The twelve earthly branches are: Zi, Chou, Yin, Mao, Chen, Si, Wu, Wei, Shen, You, Xu, and Hai. In each energy cycle, whether it is a daily, monthly, or yearly cycle, there is equivalence. A daily cycle is midnight to morning, morning to noon to the afternoon and back to midnight again. A monthly cycle is the empty moon, growing moon, full moon, and decreasing moon. A yearly cycle is spring, summer, fall, and winter. From an energetic point of view, the daily, monthly, and yearly cycles are all the same. They all have the storage, birth, growth, and decline phases.

The sages used the twelve branches to describe the similarity in these cycles. "Zi," for example, represents the state of hidden Yang energy, when it is least visible. It describes midnight, middle of winter, and an empty moon. From any particular energy cycle, Zi is where the Yang energy is least exposed or least visible. We call this phase "the storage of Yang." The earthly branch "Wu" describes Noon, middle of summer and full moon, the time where the Yang energy is most warming and most lighting.

The following is a chart of the earthly branches describing the unification of "time."

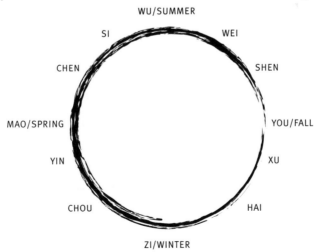

245

APPENDIX C – ACUPRESSURE POINTS

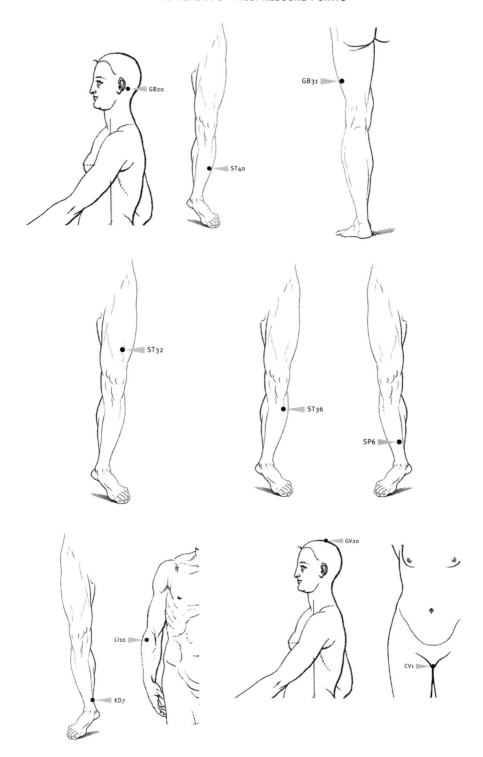

246

INDEX

247